OXFORD MEDICAL PUBL

# Risk communication and public health

# Risk communication and public health

Edited by

## Peter Bennett

*Department of Health, London, UK*

and

## Sir Kenneth Calman

*Vice Chancellor and Warden,
University of Durham, Durham, UK;
formerly Chief Medical Officer,
Department of Health, London, UK*

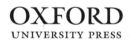

OXFORD
UNIVERSITY PRESS

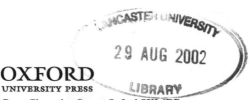

# OXFORD

UNIVERSITY PRESS

Great Clarendon Street, Oxford OX2 6DP

Oxford  New York
Athens  Auckland Bangkok  Bogota  Buenos Aires  Calcutta
Cape Town  Chennai  Dar es Salaam  Delhi  Florence  Hong Kong  Istanbul
Karachi  Kuala Lumpur  Madrid  Melbourne  Mexico City  Mumbai
Nairobi  Paris  São Paulo  Singapore  Taipei  Tokyo  Toronto  Warsaw
and associated companies in
Berlin  Ibadan

Oxford is a trade mark of Oxford University Press

Published in the United States
by Oxford University Press, Inc., New York

British Library Cataloguing in Publication Data
Data available

Library of Congress Cataloging in Publication Data
Risk communication and public health / edited by Peter Bennett and
Kenneth Calman.
(Oxford medical publications)
Includes index.
1. Health risk communication–Congresses.   2. Health risk
assessment–Congresses   3. Public health–Congresses.
4. Communication in medicine–Congresses.   I. Bennett, Peter, Dr.
II. Calman, Kenneth.   III. Series.
[DNLM: 1. Public Health congresses.   2. Risk Management
congresses.   3. Communication congresses.   WA 525 R595 1999]
RA423.2.R55   1999      362'.1–dc21      99–10437

ISBN 0 19 263037 7 (Hbk)
ISBN 0 19 850899 9 (Pbk)

Printed in Great Britain on acid free paper by
Biddles Ltd,
Guildford & King's Lynn

# Preface

> 'Decisions about risk are not technical, but value decisions'
>
> Betsy Baker
> ❖ December 1998

To those responsible for managing or regulating risks, public reactions to risk sometimes seem bizarre, at least when compared with scientific estimates. News of a hazard posing an annual risk of death of 'one chance in x' may cause near panic or virtual indifference. To the public—and particularly to those active with respect to particular issues—the behaviour of those charged with controlling risks to public health can seem no less odd. It is easy to catalogue a list of high-profile controversies about risks to public health. In the UK, prominent entries on any list will cover food safety (BSE/CJD, Listeria, Salmonella, various additives, genetic modification ...), environmental issues (air pollution, chemical discharges, radiation ...), medicines and medical treatment, (contraceptive 'pill scares', alleged vaccination risks, failures in screening programmes, 'HIV-positive surgeons' ...), 'lifestyle' risks (diet and cancer, the risks and benefits of alcohol in moderation, whether cyclists should have to wear helmets ...), and so on. On all sides, the temptation is to explain disagreements in terms of malevolence, stupidity, or both. Nor is this a peculiarly British problem. Similar cases can be cited throughout the world—while specific issues increasingly have international ramifications.

Not surprisingly then, risk *communication* is often a contentious field. Debates about health risks are seldom only about communication, but poor communication is very often a factor. From one point of view, the temptation is to see the public—egged on by the media—to be misunderstanding perfectly sensible information and advice. From the other, responsible authorities are seen to be withholding or obfuscating vital pieces of the picture and to be impervious to perfectly reasonable public concerns. Either 'the guilty' are being protected, or the public is being hectored and 'nannied' on the basis of evidence that may be overthrown tomorrow. The picture is complicated by the uncertainty that often surrounds the assessment of a particular risk, making responsible communication more difficult.

Given such controversies, it is all too easy to suppose that communication about risk is doomed to be a dialogue of the deaf. However, that is much too gloomy a view. There are plenty of cases in which—even with the benefit of hindsight—both the advice provided and the public response appear sensible enough. But what is clear is that the old-fashioned view of risk communication as a one-way process of drip-feeding expert knowledge onto a supposedly grateful public will no longer do. 'Experts' no longer command automatic deference—no matter how genuine their expertise. Increasingly, people are only prepared to listen if they feel that there is some prospect of their own views being heard.

This volume brings together a wide variety of perspectives on risk communication and public health. The 'cast list' is British, but the issues will be familiar around the world. We have been able to bring together contributors—including prominent figures in current debates about risk policy— from the public health professions, academia, campaigning organizations, think tanks, government and its independent advisory committees, and companies specializing in risk assessment and communication. The result should be of interest to:

- anyone involved in assessing and communicating about risks, whether working in the public or private sector;
- those concerned about particular risks (or possible risks) to public health, and why they do or do not seem to be taken seriously;
- students of the policy process interested in how one bit of 'the system' is responding to demands for greater openness and participation in decisions;
- those interested in the role of the media and mass communication in society, those concerned with the role of science in shaping policy, and with public perceptions of science;
- and finally, those simply wanting to understand why issues to do with possible risks to heath can generate so much controversy and ill-feeling.

The book has its origins in a conference organized by the Department of Health in November 1997. Rather than simply being a collection of papers 'as presented', however, the contributions to the book reflect both the discussion on the day and subsequent events in the world at large. We are pleased that several of the discussants have been able to provide chapters, in addition to those originally presenting papers

We concentrate on the *public* health arena, in two senses. First, we focus on the challenges of communicating with many people at once, rather than in a one-to-one setting as between doctor and patient. Nevertheless, many of the same principles also apply to both, and in some contexts—for example, following discovery of some risk of in-hospital infection—public and individual communication become intertwined. Much can depend on whether the individuals most affected feel they were kept properly informed—feelings that can shape media coverage and become a very public matter. Secondly, we are primarily concerned with risk communication as part of the *public policy process*. The material will be relevant enough to the private sector, which frequently faces its own risk communication challenges. However, government and its various arms and agencies is in a unique position of responsibility when it comes to regulating risks, setting guidelines for other authorities—e.g. in local government and the Health Service—informing citizens about risks, and generally protecting the public health. At this level, much of the debate about risk becomes interwoven with fundamental issues to do with power, information, and the relationship between people and state. Such grand questions coexist with a host of more mundane issues to do with the composition of messages and the understandings placed on words and numbers. Risk communication thus gains a unique fascination. It can also be quite literally a matter of life and death.

Each chapter in the book is self contained, but the volume is structured so as to move the discussion progressively forward.

- **Part 1** offers an introduction to risk communication as a topic of research, concentrating on findings of practical significance. Chapter 1 provides a general overview of 'what is known' from systematic research in the field, and highlights some current areas of investigation. These are taken up in more depth in Chapters 2–5, all of which report recent or ongoing empirical research.

- **Part 2** consists of studies of prominent cases and the lessons to be drawn from them. The contributions in this section look at the issues primarily from the viewpoint of those charged with regulating or controlling risks and communicating with the public.

- **Part 3** offers a series of perspectives on the wider debate about procedures and institutions.

- **Part 4** pulls together some key themes, and closes the circle by setting out their implications for those actually engaged in the process of risk communication.

In putting this volume together, we have encouraged contributors to cover those topics of most concern to them, rather than rigidly dividing the field between them. As is usual in a collection of work such as this, the views expressed are those of each contributor, and should not be taken to represent those of the editors—or, of course, the Department of Health. Though we hope to have avoided any extensive repetition, we make no apology for the fact that topics sometimes reappear, albeit from different perspectives. As a result, readers can judge the extent to which those with very different experiences and viewpoints home in on similar key themes. We believe there to be a considerable overlap of ideas on how to move forward. Controversies about risk and its communication will very properly remain, since nobody has a monopoly of wisdom. However, we are hopeful of genuine progress in raising the level of both understanding and practice.

*London*                                                    P.G.B.
*Durham*                                                    K.C.C.
*February 1999*

## Preface to the paperback edition

Since this volume originally appeared, much has happened in the world of public health. Specific issues discussed by our contributors have moved on. In the UK, the new Food Standards Agency has now formally been established. The debate on Genetic Modification of crops has become much more high-profile. The Phillips Enquiry into BSE/CJD has reported. Further research on risk and its communication has continued to appear, especially through the major programme—just concluded—on Risk and Human Behaviour sponsored by the Economic and Social Research Council. Obviously, specific facts and figures could be updated at various points. In general, however, we have been struck by how little has 'dated'. The basic messages of the various chapters seem as clear now as they first were: in general they have been vindicated rather than undermined by recent developments. We have therefore resisted any temptation to ask for revisions, though we have updated contributors' biographical details and addresses.

London                                                      PGB
Durham                                                      KCC

November 2000

# Acknowledgements

## Chapter 2

The author would like to thank the Department of Health, the Biotechnology and Biological Sciences Research Council, the Ministry of Agriculture, Fisheries and Food, and the European Commission for funding parts of the research reported.

## Chapter 3

The studies presented here were supported by a number of grants from the Economic and Social Research Council under the Global Environmental Change and Risk and Human Behaviour Programmes. The authors are very grateful to the ESRC for the financial support given.

## Chapter 4

This work is funded under a UK Department of Health contract. Thanks go to all those Environmental Health Officers and Directors of Public Health who took the time to complete the questionnaire on which this work has been based, and also to Dr Anne Spurgeon and Dr Linda Shuker for their helpful comments during the drafting of this paper. The views expressed here are those of the authors and not necessarily those of any government department or agency.

## Chapter 5

A part of the material in this paper arises from work conducted by Dr Nick Pidgeon for the Health and Safety Executive under grant No. 3625/R62.076. The opinions expressed in the chapter are, however, those of the authors alone.

## Chapter 6

I thank my secretary, Mrs Jacqueline Morrison, for meticulous record keeping, skilful handling of enquiries, and help with the analyses reported here, and the *Journal of Infection* for permission to reproduce Figures 6.1 and 6.2.

## Chapter 9

This chapter is based on a project sponsored by the following government departments: Health and Safety Executive (HSE), Department of the Environment, Transport and the Regions (DETR), Ministry of Agriculture, Fisheries and Food (MAFF), Department of Health (DH), Ministry of Defence (MoD), Treasury (HMT), and the Better Regulation Unit (BRU).

# Contents

# List of contributors

**Peter Bennett**  Department of Health, 80 London Road, London SE1 6LW

**Derek Burke**  (Former Chairman ACNFP), 13 Pretoria Road, Cambridge CB4 1HD

**David Coles**  Assistant Director, Science in Government, Office of Science and Technology, Albany House, 94–98 Petty France, London SW1H 9ST

**Anna Coote**  Director of Public Health Programme, King's Fund, 11–13 Cavendish Square, London W1M 0AN

**Sue Davies**, Consumers' Association, 2 Marylebone Road, London NW1 4DF

**Raquel Duarte-Davidson**  MRC Institute for Environment and Health, University of Leicester, 94 Regent Road, Leicester LE1 7DD

**David Fisk**  Director, Central Strategy Department of the Environment, Transport and the Regions, Directorate of Air Climate and Toxic Substances, Romney House, 43 Marsham Street, London SW1P 3YP

**Jane Franklin**  South Bank University, 103 Borough Road, London SE1 0AA

**Simon French**  Manchester Business School, University of Manchester, Booth Street, Manchester M15 6PB

**Lynn J. Frewer**  Head, Risk Perception and Communication Group, Institute of Food Research, Norwich Research Park, Colney, Norwich NR4 7UA

**Simon Gerrard**  Deputy Director, Centre of Environmental Risk, School of Environmental Sciences, University of East Anglia, Norwich NR4 7TJ

**Emma Green**  MRC Institute for Environment and Health, University of Leicester, 94 Regent Road, Leicester LE1 7DD

**Karen Henwood**  School of Health Policy and Practice, University of East Anglia, Norwich NR4 7TJ

**Ian H. Langford**  Centre for Social and Economic Research on the Global Environment, School of Environmental Sciences, University of East Anglia, Norwich NR4 7TJ

**Leonard S. Levy**  MRC Institute for Environment and Health, University of Leicester, 94 Regent Road, Leicester LE1 7DD

**Ronan A. Lyons**  Consultant in Public Health Medicine, Iechyd Morgannwg Health, 41 High Street, Swansea SA1 1LT

**Sally Macintyre**  Director, MRC Medical Sociology Unit, University of Glasgow, 6 Lilybank Gardens, Glasgow G12 8RZ

**Bryan Maguire**  School of Psychology, University of Wales, Bangor, Gwynedd LL57 2DG

**Claire Marris**  Centre d'Economie et d'Ethique pour l'Environnement et le Developpement, Universite de Versailles Saint-Quentin-en-Yvelines, France

**John Maule**  Leeds University Management School, University of Leeds, Leeds LS2 9JT

**Robert J. Maxwell**  Pitt Court Manor, N Nibley, Near Dursley, Gloucestershire GL11 6EL

**Anne McDonald**  Department of Health, 133–158 Waterloo Road, London SE1 8UG

**Sheila McKechnie**  Director, Consumers' Association, 2 Marylebone Road, London NW1 4DF

**David Miller**  Stirling Media Research Institute, University of Stirling, Stirling FK9 4LA

**Hugh Pennington**  Department of Medical Microbiology, University of Aberdeen, Aberdeen

**Nick Pidgeon**  School of Environmental Sciences, University of East Anglia, Norwich NR4 7TJ

**Timothy O'Riordan**  Centre for Social and Economic Research on the Global Environment, School of Environmental Sciences, University of East Anglia, Norwich NR4 7TJ

**Simon D. Short**   MRC Institute for Environment and Health, University of Leicester, 94 Regent Road, Leicester LE1 7DD

**Tony Taig**   Risk Solutions, 14 Upper Woburn Place, London WC1H 0JN

**Ian E. Taylor**   Scientific Political Advisor, Greenpeace UK, Canonbury Villas, Islington, London N1 2PN

**Dorothy Wright**   Deputy Director of Public Health and CCDC, Iechyd Morgannwg Health, 41 High Street, Swansea SA1 1LT

# Biographical notes

**Peter Bennett**
Dr Bennett gained a degree in Physics from Southampton University in 1972. He then studied the logic, history, and philosophy of science at Sussex University, completing an MSc in 1973, and a DPhil in 1975. He then moved to Operational Research (Management Science), initially on a research project into decision-making in conflicts. He has retained a strong interest in decisions involving conflict, risk, and uncertainty ever since, and has produced two books and over 60 research papers in this area. He moved from Sussex to Strathclyde University in 1987, serving successfully as Lecturer, Senior Lecturer, and Reader in Management Science, and as postgraduate course director. At the same time he was engaged in a number of applied research and consultancy projects, with clients ranging from international companies to local community groups. He was also highly involved in an independent group providing information and analysis on defence and foreign policy issues. In 1996 he joined the Department of Health as a principal analyst in the Economics and Operational Research Division, helping provide policy analysis on a range of topics, but with a particular emphasis on risk analysis and communication. His outside interests include music and naval history, and he is a keen dinghy sailor.

**Sir Kenneth Calman**
Sir Kenneth entered medical school in 1959. Having also taken two years out to gain an honours degree in Biochemistry, he graduated in medicine (with commendation) in 1967. During that latter part of his undergraduate medical career he developed an interest in dermatology and graduated with a PhD in 1970. Following his house jobs, he moved into the Department of Surgery in Glasgow, and proceeded to the Fellowship of the Royal College of Surgeons and an MD thesis with Honours on organ preservation. His clinical interests at this time were in general surgery, vascular surgery and transplantation. In 1972 he was the MRC Clinical Research Fellow at the Chester Beatty Research Institute in London and returned to Glasgow in 1974 as Professor of Oncology. He remained in that post for 10 years, developing particular interests in nutrition, chemotherapy, cancer education,

counselling, and patient support groups. In 1984 he became Dean of Postgraduate Medicine and Professor of Postgraduate Medical Education at the University of Glasgow, and Consultant Physician with an interest in palliative care at Victoria Infirmary, Glasgow. During this time he was involved in developing and supervising medical education projects. In 1989 he was appointed Chief Medical Officer at the Scottish Home and Health Department, and in September 1991 he became Chief Medical Officer in the Department of Health in London. He is a Fellow of numerous Royal Colleges and Faculties, and in 1979 was elected a Fellow of the Royal Society of Edinburgh. Since 1998 he has had a new role as Vice Chancellor and Warden of the University of Durham. He has written seven books and over 100 scientific papers. Sir Kenneth's outside interests include the history of medicine, Scottish literature, cartoons, and gardening. He is married with three grown-up children.

## Contributors in order of appearance

### Lynn Frewer
Dr Frewer is Head of the Risk Perception and Communication Group at the Institute of Food Research (IFR) at Norwich. Lynn graduated from the University of Bristol with a BSc in Psychology, an MSc in Economics from University College London and a PhD in applied psychology from the University of Leeds. Her current research interests include the psychology of risk perceptions and attitudes, the influence of the media on risk perceptions, public attitudes to genetic engineering, and the impact of trust on the effectiveness of risk communication.

### Ian Langford, Claire Marris, and Tim O'Riordan
Ian Langford is a Senior Research Fellow at the Centre for Social and Economic Research on the Global Environment at the University of East Anglia, and University College London. His main research interests are risk perception, epidemiology, and environmental economics. He is a Visiting Fellow at the Institute of Education, London where he is involved in research using multilevel modelling, and Visiting Lecturer at the University of the Aegean, Greece.

Claire Marris conducts social science research on risk perceptions and risk mangement. She was at the University of East Anglia from 1992 to 1996 and is currently Research Fellow at the Centre d'Economie et d'Ethique pour l'Environnement et le Developpement (C3ED) of the Universite de Versailles Saint-Quentin-en-Yvelines, France.

Professor O'Riordan is Professor of Environmental Sciences at the University of East Anglia and Associate Director of the Centre for Social and Economic Research on the Global Environment. This is jointly located at the University of East Anglia and University College, London, and is funded by the Economic and Social Research Council. Professor O'Riordan has taught and researched in Canada, where he worked for seven years in British Columbia, and in the US, Australia, and New Zealand. He is Chairman of the Broads Authority, a special statutory authority with a remit to manage the internationally important wetlands of East Anglia. He is also author of numerous books including *Environmentalism* (1981), *Sizewell B: an anatomy of the inquiry* (1987), *Controlling pollution in the Round* (1991), *Environmental science for environmental management* (1994), *Interpreting the precautionary principle* (1995), *Politics of climate change* (1996), and *Ecotaxation* (1996).

**Emma Green, Simon Short, Raquel Duarte-Davidson, and Leonard Levy**
Emma Green, Simon Short, and Leonard Levy work at the MRC Institute for Environment and Health (IEH) in Leicester. Its primary role is to rigorously assess and evaluate the links between environmental quality and human health and wellbeing. Raquel Duarte-Davidson recently moved from IEH to the National Centre for Risk Analysis and Options Appraisal at the Environment Agency.

Dr Green manages a research programme on the perception and communication of environmental risks to health as well as contributing to projects on environmental risk assessment, indoor air quality, and the regulation of pesticides in the EU.

Mr Short has also recently been examining the effects of indoor air quality in the home and is involved in research on environmental risk assessment, cost-benefit analysis, and the public's understanding of indoor air quality issues.

Dr Duarte-Davidson is responsible for establishing, maintaining, and implementing the Environment Agency's chemical pollutant risk assessment capability, ensuring that decisions are based on a credible and internationally-respected assessment of the risks of environmental and human exposures.

Dr Levy heads the Toxicology and Risk Assessment Group at IEH. His main areas of research focus on occupational and environmental toxicology and the setting of exposure limits. He has published widely on cancer, toxicology and standard setting. He is a member of the UK Advisory Committee on Toxic Substances, the Working Group on the

Assessment of Toxic Chemicals and the UK nominee on the Scientific
Committee on Exposure Limits.

**Nick Pidgeon, Karen Henwood, and Bryan Maguire**
Prof. Pidgeon is Director of the Centre for Environmental Risk, University
of East Anglia, after moving from the School of Psychology at the University of Wales Bangor. He obtained his PhD in psychology from Bristol
University in 1986 and since then has published widely on environmental
risk perception and risk communication, safety culture and organizational
learning, and on risk management. In 1991–92 he was a member of the UK
Royal Society study group on risk, and has since acted as a scientific adviser
on risk perception and communication issues to a number of UK government departments. He is presently a member of the Steering Committee of
the Economic and Social Research Council's 'Risk and human behaviour'
programme.

Dr Henwood obtained a first degree and a PhD in psychology from the
University of Bristol. She is currently Lecturer in Health and Clinical
Psychology at the School of Public Health Policy and Practice, University
of East Anglia. Her research is in the area of culture, health, and the
construction of identities, and she has also written extensively on the use
of qualitative research methods for both social and clinical scientists. She
is the editor of the book *Standpoints and differences: essays in the practice
of feminist psychology* (Sage 1998), and is currently Chair of the British
Psychological Society 'Psychology of women' section.

Dr Maguire studied psychology and pharmacology at the National University of Ireland. He was awarded his PhD by the University of California,
San Francisco for his work on health professionals' response to the HIV
epidemic. As a lecturer at the University of Wales Bangor from 1991–98
he carried out research into health professional education, educational technology, lay models of disease and decision-making by health professionals.
He is currently Head of the Department of Science at Dun Laoghaire
Institute of Art, Design and Technology in Ireland.

**Hugh Pennington**
Professor Pennington graduated in medicine and gained his PhD at St
Thomas's Hospital Medical School, London. After holding posts there and
at the Institute of Virology in Glasgow he was appointed to the Chair of
Bacteriology at Aberdeen University in 1979, a post he still holds. His
research has focused on the development of typing methods for bacteria
that cause meningitis, streptococci (the 'flesh-eating bug'), *Campylobacter*
and *E. coli* O157. He was Dean of the Medical school from 1987 to 1992 and

chaired the Pennington Group enquiry into the 1996 outbreak of *E. coli* O157 in central Scotland.

### Robert Maxwell CVO, CBE

Dr Maxwell was formerly Chief Executive of the King's Fund, retiring in 1997. He has long been interested in international comparisons of health care and health policy. His PhD (from the London School of Economics) was published in 1981 as *Health and Wealth*, an international study of health care spending. In 1997 he wrote *An Unplayable Hand? BSE, CJD and the British Government*, published by the King's Fund. He is a Trustee of the Joseph Rowntree Foundation, Vice-Chairman of the Severn NHS Trust, and chairman of the Council of the Foundation for Integrated Medicine.

### Ronan A. Lyons and Dorothy Wright

Dr Lyons is a Clinical Senior Lecturer at the Welsh Combined Centres for Public Health, University of Wales College of Medicine, a Consultant in Public Health Medicine at Iechyd Morgannwg Health, Swansea and also a Honorary Consultant in Accident and Emergency at Morriston NHS Trust, Swansea. His research interests include injury surveillance and prevention, environmental epidemiology, and health services research.

Dr Wright is the Deputy Director of Public Health and Consultant in Communicable Disease Control in Iechyd Morgannwg Health. She is Head of Emergency Planning for the Authority and was instrumental in the production of the All Wales Framework for Chemical Incidents. She is a member of the Health Authority's Risk Assessment Group.

### Tony Taig

Tony Taig is the Managing Partner of Risk Solutions, the management consulting practice of AEA Technology plc, and has had 21 years' experience in risk management and communication. He spent the early part of his career with the UK Atomic Energy Authority, where he worked on risk issues for the nuclear, chemical and transport industries, developed new applications for risk assessment and led the development of a commercial risk consulting practice within UKAEA. He spent four years in a corporate marketing and business development role before becoming one of the founding partners of Risk Solutions, set up by the newly-privatized AEA Technology in 1997. In 1997/8 he led and managed a benchmarking study of risk communication on behalf of a number of UK Government departments.

### David Fisk CB

Dr Fisk is currently Director for Central Strategy and Chief Scientist in the Department of Environment Transport and the Regions. Until 1999 he was responsible for the development of the UK Climate Change Policy (where he led the UK delegation), the UK's first National Air Quality Strategy, policy on the safe release of genetically modified organisms and chemicals onto the market, and policy on the disposal of radioactive waste. He was also responsible for the overall co-ordination of environment policy outside the European Union. He is a Fellow of the Royal Academy of Engineering, and an Honorary Fellow of the Chartered Institute of Building Services Engineers.

### Derek Burke

Professor Burke was Vice-Chancellor of the University of East Anglia from 1987–95. Before that he was Vice-President and Scientific Director of Allelix, Canada's largest biotechnology company, and Professor of Biological Sciences in the University of Warwick. He was Chairman of the Advisory Committee on Novel Foods and Processes (ACNFP) from 1988–95, and a member of the Committee on the Ethics of Genetic Modification and Food Use. He is a member of the Nuffield Council on Bioethics Working Party on Genetically Modified Crops and of the Science, Medical and Technology Committee of the Church of England's Board for Social Responsibility.

### Ian Taylor

Dr Taylor has been Scientific Political Adviser for Greenpeace UK since January 1997. This post was formed specifically to address the use and misuse of science in relation to environmental risks, with the aim of challenging environmentally detrimental uses of science and promoting beneficial applications. After graduating in Earth Sciences from Cambridge University he obtained his PhD in sedimentary geology from McMaster University Canada. Before his work with Greenpeace he worked for six years with Oxfam as a campaigner against international injustice and poverty. He has also worked in technical roles for Shell and BICC.

### Sheila McKechnie and Sue Davies

Sheila McKechnie is Director of the Consumers' Association. She has a long-standing interest in risk assessment from her involvement in occupational health and safety. CA is involved in many issues which require assessment of risk to consumers.

Sue Davies is a Principal Policy Adviser at the Consumers Association with responsibility for food issues. She is author of CA's policy report 'Confronting Risk a new approach to food safety'.

### Anna Coote and Jane Franklin

Anna Coote is a senior director at the King's Fund, London, responsible for its work on public health, inequalities and regeneration. She is a member of the London Health Commission, the Department of Health Task Force on Inequalities and Public Health, and the Sustainable Development Commission. She was formerly consultant to the Ministers for Women, Deputy Director of the Institute for Public Policy Research, editor of current affairs for Channel Four Television and Deputy Editor of the *New Statesman*. She writes widely on health and social policy.

Jane Franklin is Research Fellow and Lecturer in social policy and social theory at South Bank University, London, and was previously Research Fellow at the Institute for Public Policy Research. Her publications include, *Equality* (IPPR 1997), *The Politics of Risk Society* (Polity 1998), and 'After modernisation: gender, the third way and the new politics' in A. Coote (ed) *New Gender Agenda: why women still want more* (IPPR 2000). She is currently working for a PhD in Gender Studies at the London School of Economics.

### David Coles
Dr Coles worked as Science Policy Co-ordinator for the Department of Health, managing and co-ordinating policy on risk assessment and communication and promoting good practice on risk issues more widely through the Interdepartmental Liaison Group on Risk Assessment and other fora. After moving within the Department to take on responsibility for work on Assisted Conception, Embryology and Ethics, he was seconded to the Office of Science and Technology as Assistant Director, Sciences in Government.

### Anne McDonald
Dr McDonald has a BSc in biochemistry and an MSc in Analytical Chemistry. Following scientific posts in the Department of Health working on the health effects of food contaminants and environmental pollutants, she has a particular interest in better communication on public health risks in these areas. At the time of writing, she headed a unit working across government to develop better risk communication.

### David Miller and Sally Macintyre
David Miller works at the Stirling Media Research Centre, Stirling University.

Professor Macintyre is Director of the MRC Social and Public Health Sciences Unit at Glasgow University. A medical sociologist, she has been interested for some time in perceptions of health risks in various fields, and has collaborated on projects with media sociologists examining media coverage of a variety of topics. She has served on the Advisory Committee on Genetic Testing (ACGT) and the Advisory Group on Scientific Advances in Genetics. She is Editor-in-Chief of the International Journal *Social Science and Medicine*.

**Simon French and John Maule**

Professor French works in the Business School of Manchester University and has interests in the impacts of information and communication technologies, particularly those relating to risk and decision support. He was a member of the International Chernobyl Project and is heavily involved in European research programmes to manage future emergencies better.

Dr Maule is Senior Lecturer in Management Decision Making at Leeds University Business School. He is a psychologist currently researching the effects of mood, emotion, and time pressure on decision making, how people model risk in strategic decisions, and informed decision-making by patients. He has wide experience of teaching professional groups how to improve their decision-making through better ways of reasoning and the use of structured decision aids.

**Simon Gerrard**

Dr Gerrard is Deputy Director of the Centre for Environmental Risk at the University of East Anglia, Norwich. The Centre is a research organization based within the School of Environmental Sciences specializing in environment and health risk assessment, perception, communication, and management.

# PART 1

Research perspectives: what do we know and where are the frontiers?

# 1 Understanding responses to risk: some basic findings

Peter Bennett
*Department of Health, London*

## Introduction

What is actually known about how we react to risks, and to messages about them? While much remains to be fully understood, research has uncovered some helpful findings. This chapter attempts a critical review of this literature—necessarily in broad-brush terms—so as to provide a starting point for further discussion. We comment briefly on some practical implications for risk communication, points taken up more fully in Part IV of the book. The chapters making up the rest of Part I explore some of the research in more detail and outline current work. They also provide more detailed references, those given here being confined to a few key works on each topic.

To start with a general point, there has been a progressive change in the literature on risk:

- *from* an emphasis on 'public *misperceptions*', with a tendency to treat all deviations from expert estimates as products of ignorance or stupidity
- *via* empirical investigation of what actually concerns people and why
- *to* approaches which stress that public reactions to risk often have a rationality of their own, and that 'expert' and 'lay' perspectives should inform each other as part of a two-way process.

For risk communication, research under the second and third headings offers some key insights. An appreciation of what causes concern may allow some forward planning rather than continual crisis management. Treating communication as a two-way process, if taken seriously, has profound consequences for the whole business of risk assessment and regulation. This is not to deny that public misunderstandings exist: people may sometimes be most frightened by the 'wrong' hazards. So research on misperceptions, though maybe less fashionable, still offers some valuable insights—particularly applied without any presumption that misperceptions affect *only* 'the public'. There is good evidence to suggest that everyone—including scientists, regulators, politicians, journalists, and members of the public—is prone to bias in the use of information, *particularly* when it comes to processing probabilities. Not only is everyone dealing with risk fallible: we are fallible in some predictable directions. Once this is appreciated, one can begin to design processes to mitigate the consequences.

If scientific and lay perspectives are to inform each other, those responsible for communicating about risks have both to take public concerns seriously while still doing justice to available scientific evidence. This can be a difficult balancing act. As argued in subsequent chapters, very often answers have to be found in the *process* of communication and engagement with relevant stakeholders, rather than just the fine-tuning of words. The rest of this chapter introduces some findings that can help underpin better practice, as well as being of interest in their own right. They are summarized under the following headings:

- trust
- risk perceptions
- risk and values
- risk comparisons
- understanding probability
- indirect effects and the social amplification of risks.

In each case, this chapter concentrates on points that seem fairly well established. Some continuing debates are noted in passing, with references to more in-depth discussion later in the book.

# Trust

Perhaps surprisingly, the role of trust in risk communication is a comparatively recent focus for systematic research. Nevertheless, trust is a logical topic with which to start, as its presence or absence conditions all other aspects of communication (Renn and Levine 1991). Put simply, the point is that messages are often judged first and foremost not by content but by source: *who is telling me this, and can I trust them*? If the answer to the second question is 'no', *any* message from that source will often be disregarded, no matter how well intentioned and well delivered. Indeed, good delivery may even be counter-productive. There is some evidence that well-presented arguments from distrusted sources have a negative effect—as if people conclude that the sender is not only untrustworthy but cunning as well.

It is not hard to find studies featuring the government being seen as an untrustworthy source (specific survey findings are cited in Chapters 2, 3, and 13). Industry sources are often seen as biased, even if competent. Medical doctors start with a much higher level of credibility, but reactions to high-profile incidents (e.g. 'HIV-positive surgeons') show how fragile even this can be. There are no known ways of generating instant trust, even when deserved. However, the literature does offer some strong clues as to how trust is won or lost. Three are worth noting at this stage:

1.  First, actions often do speak louder than words: organizational 'body language' is important. Appearing to act only under pressure, for example, can be fatal. This applies not only to how the organization acts relative to the case in hand, but also to the overall impression people have of it. Messages deliberately sent are usually only a minor part of the overall message conveyed.

2.  Trust is generally reinforced by 'openness', not only in the sense of making information available, but in giving a candid account of the evidence underlying decisions and how it was used.

3.  Studies repeatedly show that the response to a message depends not only on its content but also on the manner of delivery. An important component of manner is *emotional tone*: for example, to engage with an outraged audience it is first necessary to acknowledge the outrage.

Research has also shown trust to be multifaceted rather than one-dimensional. Relevant factors include perceived competence, objectivity, fairness, consistency, and goodwill; particular sources may score differently on these dimensions, and across different issues. For example, there is evidence of both the Department of Health and the Department of the Environment being rather *highly* trusted when it comes to radiological safety—in fact more so than environmental campaigners (Hunt *et al.* 1998). Questions about who is trusted may be intertwined with questions about who should be held to account for particular risk problems. These issues are discussed more fully in Chapters 2 and 3, and reappear at many other points below. It also seems that statements about trust may not match actual responses to messages: for example, people may *say* they distrust the government yet be greatly influenced by government statements (see Chapter 18). For the present, the important point is that black-and-white judgements are not inevitable. There are plenty of cases in which a fair degree of trust has been maintained even in difficult circumstances. However, there is strong evidence that if trust *is* lost, re-establishing it is a long and uphill task.

# Risk perceptions: 'fright factors'

Why do some risks trigger so much more alarm, anxiety, or outrage than others, seemingly regardless of scientific estimates of their seriousness? Research over many years in the so-called 'psychometric' tradition (Fischhoff *et al.* 1978, 1991; Slovic 1986; Gardner and Gould 1989) has sought to find answers to this key question. From this have emerged some fairly well-established rules of thumb. These may be summarized by the 'fright factors' shown in Box 1.1.

---

**Box 1.1: Fright factors**

---

Risks are generally more worrying (and less acceptable) if perceived:

1. To be **involuntary** (e.g. exposure to pollution) rather than voluntary (e.g. dangerous sports or smoking).
2. As **inequitably distributed** (some benefit while others suffer the consequences).
3. As **inescapable** by taking personal precautions.
4. To arise from an **unfamiliar or novel** source.
5. To result from **man-made, rather than natural** sources.
6. To cause **hidden and irreversible** damage, e.g. through onset of illness many years after exposure.
7. To pose some particular danger to **small children or pregnant women** or more generally to **future generations**.
8. To threaten a form of death (or illness/injury) **arousing particular dread**.
9. To damage **identifiable rather than anonymous victims**.
10. To be **poorly understood by science**.
11. As subject to **contradictory statements** from responsible sources (or, even worse, from the same source).

---

The fright factors attempt to combine the most significant items from several extant lists. Terminology varies somewhat, e.g. some authors group several factors together under the label 'dread', which is used in a narrower sense here. Lest the results seem too cut-and-dried, debate remains as to which particular factors are most important, for whom, and for what issues (much of the underlying research is US-based, and attitudes toward nuclear power over-represented). Strictly speaking, the separate factors are also interdependent rather than additive. For example, if no other fright factors are present, the last two may invite the blasé response 'anything *might* be risky, so why worry about this?'. Nevertheless, there is little disagreement that factors of this type are important much of the time. One consequence is that statistics on risk will never be all-important. Nevertheless, reactions to risk are not entirely arbitrary. The list just given can be used as a diagnostic checklist and—perhaps with more difficulty—as an aid to prediction.

# Risk and values

Though fright factors may distort perceptions by highlighting certain types of risk, there is no basis for dismissing them as unreasonable *per se*. They may, in fact, reflect defensible *value judgements*. Risk of death by cancer, for example, usually carries much greater dread than the prospect of a sudden heart attack. Given the inevitability of death itself, it would be perverse to regard this as irrational. Similarly, willingness to accept voluntary risks may reflect the value placed on personal autonomy. Indeed, risk often has attractions: mountaineers, hang-gliders and racing drivers take precautions to limit the risks they take, but facing *some* risk is undeniably part of the fun. The general point is that responses to risk are not only dependent on context, but intertwined with personal values—a point well argued in the popular book by Adams (1995). Attitudes to specific risks are influenced by beliefs about how society is and should be, our relationship with nature, the benefits and disadvantages of technology, etc.—not to mention religious belief. All will help determine which fright factors most frighten and what sources (and forms) of information are trusted.

Given that people's value systems and personalities differ, it should come as no surprise to learn that while the fright factors are quite good indicators of the overall public response to risks, they are only weak predictors of how any *individual* will react. The latter can depend strongly on approval or disapproval of an activity on other grounds. Those who love (or hate) the motor car anyway usually entertain smaller (or greater) estimates of its health risks. Similarly, debates about nuclear power are about more than just risk, or even 'risk plus fright factors'. (As with the claim that achieving 'technical' safety—even if feasible—would require an unacceptably authoritarian society. The point here is not to pass judgement on such views, but to note their relevance.) At the other end of the scale, emphasizing the dangers of drug abuse will have no effect on those who relish personal risk any more than teenagers playing chicken on the railway line will be deterred by the sober revelation that it is dangerous. Otherwise, why bother to play?

Some attempts have been made to categorize general attitudes to risk. For example, Cultural Theory distinguishes egalitarian, individualist, hierarchist, and fatalist world-views. *Egalitarians* tend to see the balance of nature as fragile, to distrust expertise, and strongly favour public participation in decisions. *Individualists* want to make their own decisions, and see nature as relatively robust. *Hierarchists* want well-established rules and procedures to regulate risks, while *fatalists* see such life as capricious and attempts at control as futile. Each will react to risks in different ways. The typology is set out more fully in Chapter 3. As noted there, the theory is not without its critics, and predicting individual responses to specific risks remains elusive. Recent developments of Cultural Theory recognize that people seldom conform *consistently* to any of the four ideal types. Most of us are capable of thinking in different ways: we may unconsciously put on individualist, hierarchist, egalitarian, or fatalist 'spectacles'. This recognition may make the theory richer, but unfortunately weakens its predictive power, unless and until more is known about what triggers these mental responses.

## Risk comparisons

Many efforts at risk communication offer comparative data on different risks, e.g. juxtaposing the risk of death from an air pollutant with that from smoking a single cigarette, or driving 100 miles, etc. Sometimes these comparisons have been put together to make risk 'scales' or 'ladders' (Paling 1997). The rationale for this approach is two-fold. The first point is simply that small probabilities are very difficult to conceptualize: just how small, in practical terms, is 'a risk of 1 in $10^6$', or 'a probability of 0.00015'? Numerical comparisons between different risks might help. Secondly, one result of the psychometric research outlined earlier has been to 'calibrate' public perceptions of risk against 'real' data, in particular mortality statistics. Figure 1.1 shows a typical example. Such studies repeatedly show a general over-estimation of death due to unusual or dramatic causes (floods, tornados, rare diseases) and an under-estimation of common killers such as heart disease. This demonstrates what psychologists know as the *availability bias*: the tendency to judge probability by how easily examples can be brought to mind produces distortions if certain events are highly memorable or newsworthy. So another aim of risk comparisons is often to correct this bias.

Although such findings are well established, their implications have been hotly debated. Some writers have used them to 'prove' the public's inability to make sensible judgements about risks. However, this interpretation is now largely discredited (Freudenburg and Pastor 1992). Although the perceived estimates are quantitatively biased, they do generally match the actual ordering of deaths from more to less common. More importantly, expert judgements turn out to be prone to very similar biases. Mismatches against the statistics may also reflect different interpretations of the concept of risk, e.g. those more alarmed by involuntary dangers will tend to describe these as riskier.

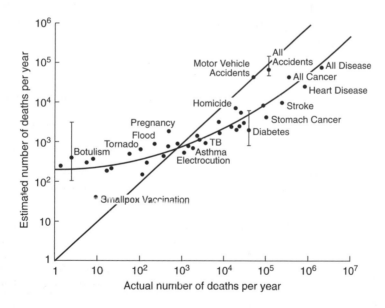

**Fig. 1.1** Estimated and actual frequency of deaths from various causes. (From Fischhoff *et al.* (1981).) Data points show the averaged responses of a sample of US population. If estimated and actual frequencies agreed, the data would lie on the straight line shown, rather than roughly following the curve. Note that both scales on the graph are logarithmic: i.e. each division makes the risk ten times greater or smaller.

To return to risk comparisons as an aid to communication, a typical example is shown in Table 1.1. Introducing a common yardstick—the 'one in a million' chance of death—is certainly thought-provoking. Nevertheless, such comparisons have acquired a very checkered reputation. Because they typically omit both the effects of fright factors and the values of the audience, they often miss the point. The example shown here—which is both widely cited and more informative than many of its kind—can be criticized for juxtaposing voluntary and involuntary risks and wildly different forms of death (accident, cancer). Furthermore, the numbers can give a false impression of precision. There is no indication that the figures may be highly uncertain (e.g. studies of toxicity loosely derived from animal data), hotly contested (nuclear power!) or both. Where, the sceptic may ask, do the figures come from, and why should I trust them?

Comparisons between risks are not *always* unhelpful, though it remains far from clear when they will 'work' (Roth *et al.* 1990). However, one essential distinction is between using comparisons simply to provide a sense of perspective and using them to imply acceptability—'you are irrational to worry about *this* risk when you happily accept *that* greater one'. Implying acceptability (or unacceptability) is at best a dubious exercise. One cannot stop people searching out figures to prove a point, but responsible use of comparative figures requires careful thought.[1]

**Table 1.1**   Examples of risks 'estimated to increase the annual chance of death by one in one million'

| Activity Cause of death | |
|---|---|
| Smoking 1.4 cigarettes | Cancer, heart disease |
| Spending 1 hour in a coal mine | Black lung disease |
| Living 2 days in New York or Boston | Air pollution |
| Travelling 10 miles by bicycle | Accident |
| Flying 1000 miles by jet | Accident |
| Living 2 months in Denver (rather than New York) | Cancer (cosmic radiation) |
| One chest X-ray in a good hospital | Cancer (from radiation) |
| Eating 40 tablespoons of peanut butter | Liver cancer (aflatoxin B) |
| Drinking 30 12-oz cans of diet soda | Cancer (from saccharin) |
| Living 150 years within 20 miles of nuclear power plant | Cancer (from radiation) |

Source: Wilson 1979.

1. In the UK, the recent ban of beef on the bone has prompted a rash of media articles comparing the risk from new variant Creutzfeldt-Jacob Disease with that of being struck by lightning, choking to death on one's steak, and so on, blithely ignoring all the above points. In this case, the aim seems to be to 'prove' that the government and its advisors are stupid, rather than the public.

# Understanding probability

## Heuristics and biases

Risk is essentially to do with chance—an unpleasant outcome is possible, but how likely is it? The accepted measure of likelihood is probability, and probabilities obey well-known mathematical laws. However, the human brain tends to manipulate them in ways that can ignore this logic, and sometimes contradict it. The problem is not so much lack of intelligence as ingrained patterns of thought—simplified ways of managing information (or *heuristics*)—that serve well enough in most situations, but give misleading results in others. Left unchecked, they lead to various common biases in dealing with probabilities (Tversky and Kahneman 1974; Dawes 1988). As these are not discussed at length elsewhere in this volume, it is worth setting out some of the most relevant here.

1. One already noted is the *availability bias*: events are perceived to be more frequent if we can easily recall examples of them. This leads us to overestimate the frequency of memorable events, and hence the chance of something similar happening again.

2. Another is *confirmation bias*: once we have formed a view, new evidence is generally made to fit: contrary information is typically filtered out, ambiguous information interpreted as confirmation, and consistent information seen as 'proof positive'. Hence views can become virtually impervious to disproof. We also often act in ways that make expectations self-fulfilling.

3. Not surprisingly then, *overconfidence* is another common feature. We are generally 'poorly calibrated' in judging the probability of being correct. Someone whose predictions in a given area are right 60% of the time should express '60% confidence' in them. But the latter figure is typically higher. Overconfidence has been widely investigated, and appears to affect almost all professions, scientific or otherwise, as well as the lay public. The few exceptions are those who receive constant feedback on the accuracy of their predictions. Weather forecasters may not be the most accurate predictors, but they are unusually well calibrated!

4. There are also problems with how separate probabilities are combined. One of particular importance is illustrated in Boxes 1.2a and 1.2b (diagnosing Blenkinsop's Syndrome). The reader might like to use this hypothetical example as a 'self-test'.

---

**Box 1.2a: Diagnosing Blenkinsop's Syndrome**

---

Blenkinsop's Syndrome is a particularly nasty disease affecting 2% of the population. Once symptoms have developed, it is generally too late for effective treatment, and death can be slow and painful. If caught early, there is an effective cure. The problem is that at that stage there are no warning symptoms.

Fortunately a test for Blenkinsop's has been developed, and a screening programme is in place. The test is a good one, in that anyone with the disease will show test positive (there are no 'false negatives'), while 90% of those without the disease will test negative.

**Someone has just tested positive for Blenkinsop's. What is the chance that they actually have the disease?**

---

The answer is given, and explained, in Box 1.2b. Many people find it surprising. The example illustrates how baseline probabilities are often ignored —or at least given insufficient weight. Avoiding this bias is particularly important when risks increase or decrease. Responses can depend critically on whether the relevant probabilities are expressed in *absolute* terms ('the chance was 2% and is now 3%') or *relative* terms (as in 'the chance has gone up by a factor of . . .' or 'this group suffers ten times the normal risk of . . .'). Relative risks sound newsworthy, but can be seriously misleading if the baseline risk is not clear. To illustrate, suppose 10 million people are exposed to two fatal risks. News that Risk A has doubled may sound much more alarming than B increasing by 10%. But if the baseline probabilities of death from A and B are 1 in $10^8$ and 1 in $10^4$ respectively, doubling A produces one extra fatality, while the 'smaller' increase in B kills 100.

## Framing effects

In reacting to probability and risk, it is often possible to 'frame' the situation in different ways, in terms of how the available information is mentally arranged. In contrast to the biasing effects just noted, this does not necessarily lead to erroneous conclusions, but different ways of framing certainly lead to different conclusions.

Probably the most common example is that outcomes may be measured against different presumed starting points (as with the bottle half-full or half-empty). The possible impact can be demonstrated experimentally by

---

**Box 1.2b: Blenkinsop's revisited**

---

The correct answer is about 17%, i.e. just over a *one-in-six* chance. Most people arrive at much more pessimistic answers, estimates of well over 50% being common. What is happening here is that too much attention is being paid to the reliability of the test (the 90%) and not enough to the baseline probability of 2% for the disease.

The mathematics of combining probabilities is governed by Bayes' Theorem. More simply, the answer in this case can be explained as follows:

Consider 1000 people taking the test. On average 20 of them will actually have Blenkinsop's, and all will test positive. Of the other 980, we should expect 10% to test positive without having the disease. There will thus be 98 false positives. Is someone testing positive one of the 20 true positives, rather than one of the 98 false ones? The chance is 20 in 118, or 16.9%.

The need to overcome such biases is common not only in medical diagnosis but in many other contexts. The tendency is to pay too much attention to indicators and not enough to underlying baseline probabilities. An additional problem is worth mentioning. In the example, it was supposed that the base probability is actually known (by some independent measure such as the number of people eventually developing clinical symptoms). In reality, this may not be the case. Repeated 'supposed-positive' results might convince people that the disease is actually quite common. One would therefore have an exaggerated idea of the base rate, making subsequent positive tests look even more convincing.

---

presenting the same decision problem in different ways. A typical study (McNeil *et al.* 1982) presented people with a hypothetical choice between two cancer therapies with different probabilities of success and failure. Half were told about the relative chances of dying while the rest had the *same* information presented in terms of survival rates. This more than doubled the numbers choosing one alternative. Perhaps most strikingly, the effect was just as great for physicians as for the general public. Similar studies show consistent results. As with gamblers who bet more wildly to recoup losses, people tend to make riskier choices if all alternatives are framed in terms of possible losses, but play safe if choosing between alternative gains. Of course, neither way of looking at the problem is 'wrong'.

More generally, it is worth reiterating that people can approach risks from completely different frames of reference, and hence define the issues in very different terms. If a regulator sets some allowable maximum level for an industrial pollutant, is it protecting the public from a risk, or legitimising one? People may, indeed, perceive different sorts of decision—for example some may presume that they are engaged in a negotiation, while others see only the search for the best technical solution.

## Scientific and lay perspectives

One particular difference in framing that bedevils risk communication is that between a 'natural science' perspective on risk and that typically held by a lay audience. Overcoming this is not merely a matter of explaining the science in lay terms—important though this is. Arguably the most important difference is that scientists usually define risk in terms of effects on populations, while the lay audience is concerned with effects on individuals.[2] Though both may be couched in terms of probability, this can disguise very different uses of the term. On the one hand lie statements about the incidence of a disease, and whether a pollutant causes any significant variation. On the other is the stark question 'what is the chance of this making *me* ill?'. Some will deny the difference by arguing that the latter question can only be answered in statistical terms. The communication problem then becomes one of educating the populace. However, there are logical—not just psychological—difficulties here. It is not necessarily valid to make a direct inference from group statistics to the risks facing individuals (Walker 1995). To do so is to assume both that the individual is entirely representative of the population—has *no* relevant distinguishing features—and that the distribution of risk is truly random. Neither will be literally true, though they may be fair approximations.

---

2. Chapter 3 makes the point that there may also be important differences regarding the burden of proof in establishing cause and effect. Another frequently cited difference is that the public is scared by the possibility of catastrophe, while scientists are more reassured by low probabilities. This has some plausibility in the context of hostile responses to the siting of power stations and other 'LULUs' (Locally Unwanted Land Uses). But in other contexts people may be *unduly* reassured by long odds—e.g. in ignoring advice on 'safe sex'. Such apparent contradictions may again be understood if people have other reasons for antagonism or enthusiasm toward the source of the risk. There is also a need for more empirical research on which risks actually concern the 'experts' in a given field as compared with the lay public. This topic is addressed in Chapter 4.

The lay perspective is more likely to start from the presumption that 'the average person does not exist'. If the statistics can be broken down to show how a risk depends on age, sex, place of work, lifestyle, and so on, the gap between the perspectives narrows. Even so, individuals may feel they escape such classifications. For example, personal experience may suggest that one is very sensitive to certain pollutants, and hence at greater risk.[3] Given that sensitivity can indeed vary widely, it would be rash to dismiss such beliefs. The problem is that science necessarily deals with reproducible effects and controlled conditions; from the opposite perspective, this can look merely artificial.

Finally, it is also noteworthy that two quite different notions of probability have currency even within science (Lilford and Braunholtz 1996). Traditional methods define probability in terms of *relative frequency* of events. However, these have increasingly been challenged by 'subjective' (or Bayesian) methods in which probability means *degree of belief*—an idea perhaps closer to the lay understanding of probability. In most circumstances, the two approaches give the same numerical results, but not always. Even if the numbers are not in dispute, different interpretations can cause confusion. If a scientist refers to a 'one in a million' probability of suffering illness X as a result of Y, he/she may mean that 'evidence suggests that Y will cause about one extra case of X per million population'. The scientist may or may not attach a high degree of certainty to the estimate. To a lay audience, the message may be heard as 'I am extremely confident—virtually certain—that you will not get X as a result of Y'. This would be a very different claim.

# Indirect effects and the 'social amplification' of risk

Events to do with risk can be likened to a stone dropping in a pool. Sometimes there is little more than the initial splash; sometimes the ripples spread far and wide. In many cases the indirect effects—caused, as it were, by the distant ripples—can far exceed the direct ones. This is most obvious with events such as accidents: it has been remarked that although 'no-one died' at Three Mile Island, the nuclear malfunction there had huge indirect effects on the industry worldwide. Sometimes an event gains significance not so much because of what has happened, but because of what it seems to portend. A classic example is seen in the *New Yorker* editorial of 18 February 1985 on the Bhopal disaster:

---

3. Conversely, health promotion efforts (e.g. on smoking) may be undermined by an 'optimistic bias', in which individuals deny that the statistics apply to them (see Chapter 2). However, the empirical evidence on this is less clear-cut than is often supposed, and it may be more helpful to consider how responses to advice differ between individuals.

'What truly grips us ... is not so much the numbers as the spectacle of suddenly vanishing competence, of men utterly routed by technology, of fail-safe systems failing with a logic as inexorable as it was once—indeed, right up to that very moment—unforeseeable. And the spectacle haunts us because it seems to carry allegorical import, like the whispery omen of a hovering future'.

Such an event can be seen not as a localized problem but as a signal or harbinger of general doom—e.g. that assurances about safety are always untrustworthy, or that 'we will regret playing with nature'. What is less clear is why some events acquire such significance, out of all those that *could* do so. Risk communication can itself have its own indirect effects. If a health warning is issued on a prominent variety of cheese or wine, rival producers may rejoice at first. But their glee is typically cut short as they find that consumers also ('unfairly!') shun *their* products. They may be forced to close or to lay off staff, with further indirect effects. Then there may be expensive attempts to restore confidence, political recriminations—perhaps international in scope—and so on.

As to when these effects are most pronounced, the factors noted before will again be relevant. However, additional features come into play once we consider the social system rather than only individual perceptions. Theories have been proposed to categorize and explain how social processes amplify—or sometimes attenuate—the effects of risk (Kasperson *et al.* 1988; Krimsky and Golding 1992). This field is reviewed more fully in Chapter 5. The mass media clearly play a major role here. Reportage affects both perceptions of risk in general, and how specific issues are initially framed. Then as an episode develops, reports of people's reactions to the original risk feed the indirect effects. Many specific examples are discussed in other chapters, particularly in Part II of the book, and some general conclusions are offered in Chapter 18. As it also points out, however, the mass media are not all-important. Professional (e.g. medical/scientific) networks are often also significant, as are informal networks of friends and acquaintances—the classic 'grapevine'. People typically trust the goodwill of family and friends more than any institutional source, while access to decentralized media such as the Internet seems set to increase the influence of self-organized networks. In any case, to blame 'sensationalist reporting' for exaggerated fears is largely to miss the point. Media coverage may well amplify the public's interest in dramatic forms of mishap, but it does not create it. A 'good story' is one in which public and media interest reinforce each other. It is difficult to see how this could be otherwise.

The question of why some particular stories about health risks 'take off' spectacularly is the subject of continuing research. Alongside the fright factors already noted, the media triggers listed in Box 1.3 provide additional (though less thoroughly-researched) indicators.

---

**Box 1.3: Media triggers**

---

A possible risk to public health is more likely to become a major story if the following are prominent or can readily be made to become so:

1. Questions of **blame**.
2. Alleged **secrets and attempted cover-ups**.
3. **Human interest** through identifiable heroes, villains, dupes, etc. (as well as victims).
4. Links with **existing high-profile issues or personalities**.
5. **Conflict**.
6. **Signal value**: the story as a portent of further ills ('*What next?*').
7. **Many people exposed** to the risk, even if at low levels ('*It could be you!*').
8. Strong **visual impact** (e.g. pictures of suffering).
9. Links to **sex** and/or **crime**.

---

Of the triggers listed, there is some evidence that the single most important is *blame*, particularly in keeping a story running for a long period. However, each case may be affected by many factors, including chance (e.g. a shortage or glut of competing stories). Once a story is established, the very fact that there is interest in the topic becomes a related story. The result can be that reportage 'snowballs' as media compete for coverage. Stories also sometimes have an 'incubation period': interest can erupt some time after the actual event, catching out the unwary.

# Final comments

The aim of this chapter has been to provide a fairly rapid tour of risk communication as a research field. As readers already familiar with the area will appreciate, coverage has been by no means exhaustive, nor has it been possible to do justice to the subtleties of the work covered. Nevertheless, an appreciation of the basic points covered here should be helpful to anyone interested in the challenges of effective risk communication, and will also serve as a baseline for more in-depth discussion in following chapters.

## REFERENCES

Adams, J. (1995). *Risk*. University College London Press, London.

Dawes, R. L. (1988). *Rational choice in an uncertain world*. Harcourt Brace, Orlando.

Fischhoff, B., Slovic, P., Lichtenstein, S., Read, S., and Coombes, B. (1978). How safe is safe enough? A psychometric study of attitudes towards technological risks and benefits. *Policy Sciences*, **9**, 127–52.

Fischhoff, B., Lichtenstein, S., Slovic, P., Derby, S. L., and Keeney, R. L. (1981). *Acceptable risk*. Cambridge University Press, Cambridge.

Freudenburg, W. R. and Pastor, S. K. (1992). NIMBYs and LULUs: Stalking the syndromes. *Journal of Social Issues*, **48**, 39–61.

Gardner, G. T. and Gould, L. C. (1989). Public perceptions of the risks and benefits of technology. *Risk Analysis*, **9**, 225–42.

Hunt, S., Frewer, L. J., and Shepherd, R. (1998). *Public trust in sources of information about radiation risks*. Institute of Food Research Report.

Kasperson, R.E. *et al*. (1988). the social amplification of risk: a conceptual framework. *Risk Analysis*, **8**, 177–87.

Krimsky, S. and Golding, D. (ed.) (1992). *Societal theories of risk*. Praeger, New York.

Lilford, R. J. and Braunholtz, D. (1996). The statistical basis of public policy; a paradigm shift is overdue. *British Medical Journal*, 7 Sept, 603–7.

McNeil, B. J., Pauker, S.G., Sox, H.C., and Tversky, A. (1982). On the elicitation of preferences for alternative therapies. *New England Journal of Medicine*, **306**, 1259–62.

Paling, J. (1997). *Up to your armpits is alligators? How to sort out what risks are worth worrying about*. Risk Communication and Environmental Institute, Gainesville.

Renn, O. and Levine, D. (1991). Credibility and trust in risk communication. In *Communicating risks to the public: international perspectives* (ed. R. E. Kasperson and P. J. M. Stallen). Kluwer, Dordrecht.

Roth, E. *et al*. (1990). What do we know about making risk comparisons? *Risk Analysis*, **10**, 375–87.

Slovic, P. (1986). Informing and educating the public about risk. *Risk Analysis*, **6**, 403–15.

Tversky, A. and Kahneman, D. (1974). Judgement under uncertainty: heuristics and biases. *Science*, **185**, 1124–31.

Walker, V. R. (1995). Direct inference, probability, and a conceptual gap in risk communication, risk analysis. *Risk Analysis,* **15**, 603–9.

Wilson, R. (1979). Analysing the daily risks of life. *Technology Review*, **81**, 40–6, 403–15.

# 2 Public risk perceptions and risk communication

Lynn J. Frewer
*Institute of Food Research, Norwich Research Park, Norwich*

## Public risk perceptions and hazard differentiation

Risk perceptions are socially constructed, and individual behaviours are driven by perceptions or beliefs about risks, and not the technical risk estimates provided by experts. It is important to examine the wider social context in which different hazards, and risk information provided about those hazards, is embedded. The psychometric approach developed by Slovic and his co-workers (Fischhoff *et al.* 1978) has indicated that factors such as whether the risk is perceived as involuntary, whether it will affect large numbers of people, or is seen to be unnatural are likely to be important determinants of public responses, and partly explain the disparity between lay and expert beliefs about risks (Flynn *et al.* 1993). This approach has generally been referred to as the psychometric paradigm in the risk perception literature.

The psychometric paradigm is regarded as an extremely important starting point for understanding risk perceptions and how the public makes decisions regarding risk mitigation priorities. However, there are a number of potentially problematic assumptions and limitations associated with the psychometric paradigm:

1. It assumes that people can provide meaningful answers to difficult, if not impossible, questions (e.g. what is the risk of death in the US from nuclear power).

2. The results are dependent upon the set of hazards studied, the questions asked about these hazards, the types of persons questioned, and the data analysis methods.

3. The questions typically assess cognitions, not actual behaviour.

Clearly risk communication is likely to be more effective if it addresses the actual concerns of the public regarding a particular hazard, not just those concerns which are believed to be important by experts. Extrapolating from this, methods must be devised that enable individuals to describe their concerns using their own terminology, to avoid the problems associated with the imposition of risk characteristics upon individuals by the researchers conducting the experiment.

Other psychological effects, such as 'optimistic bias' or 'unreal optimism' (Weinstein 1980), where people tend to believe they are less at risk from a given hazard relative to an 'average' member of society, or indeed compared to someone else with similar demographic characteristics, may represent a barrier to effective risk communication, as individuals will tend to perceive that risk information is directed towards other people who are more at risk. The actual impact that such optimistic biases have on lifestyle decisions merits further investigation, as there is little research demonstrating behavioural effects resulting from optimistic biases. In addition, the underlying psychological determinants of personal risk may be very different to perceptions of risk to the average person, and these need to be understood before the causes and likely effects of optimistic bias can be truly understood and effective risk communications developed. For example, for food risks, optimistic biases are much greater for lifestyle hazards than for those associated with the technologies involved in food production (Frewer *et al.* 1994). Even for different lifestyle hazards, there are differences in optimistic bias effects which are influenced by perceptual characteristics of the different hazards. For example, research into risk communication about microbiological risk is less dependent on source characteristics than other types of food hazard. A social psychological model of attitude change, the elaboration likelihood model, was adapted to investigate the potential impact of information source characteristics and persuasive content of information on people's engagement in elaborative, or thoughtful, cognitions about risk messages. The effects of source credibility, persuasive content of information, and hazard type were systematically varied within the model. The impact of the different factors on beliefs about the information and elaborative processing of message content was then examined. For microbiological risks, source characteristics had little effect, although this was not true for communication about alcohol use. The major barrier to effective communication about microbiological risks appeared to be the effect of optimistic bias, whereas source characteristics were more important in determining the effects of communication about alcohol (Frewer *et al.* 1997*b*).

Lifestyle risks (over which the individual has a high degree of perceived personal control) may be discounted as being less threatening to the self, but more threatening to other people, because of the need for high personal control in maintaining a positive self image. The reduction in optimistic bias for technological food hazards probably reflects the perception that personal control of the hazard is not possible, and that risk must therefore be equitably spread across the population. In the case of technological hazards, personal risk perceptions are likely to be very much linked to trust in those responsible for regulating the risks, both from the perspective of competence to control the risk in an appropriate way, and prioritizing public welfare through appropriate risk mitigation actions. However, risk estimates obtained from individuals living close to local power plants have been reported as being lower than for those individuals living elsewhere, implying that cognitive processes of risk reduction can apply even to hazards over which individuals have very little personal control (Van der Pligt *et al.* 1986). Furthermore, the 'illusion of knowledge', where people tend to think that they know more about the hazard than other people, will tend to result in individuals assuming the information is directed towards others who are more ignorant about the risks (Frewer *et al.* 1994).

It is also important to examine the actual numbers of people exhibiting optimistic bias effects in the population studied. Not all individuals may exhibit optimistic biases, and the percentage of people who do may vary across different types of hazard. Simply examining average scores for personal and general risk perceptions for the population sampled may obscure these individual differences.

It is essential to attempt to understand what type of psychological factors are driving people's risk perceptions. It becomes necessary to use new methodological techniques, such as semi-structured interviewing, in conjunction with statistical methods aimed at examining the extent to which people agree about their underlying concerns associated with particular hazards. Experimental work utilizing this type of methodology has shown that:

1.  Public concerns are very often specific to a particular hazard domain. For example, in the case of genetic engineering, ethical concerns dominate issues of public concern, and cannot be dissociated from risk communication issues (Frewer *et al.* 1997c).

2.  Perceptions of benefit or need may offset perceptions of risk in the context of public decision-making regarding acceptability (Frewer *et al.*, 1998a).

Indeed, it is possible that people are more concerned about the extent of the benefits resulting from the development and application of a particular technology than the associated risks. As long as a risk is not so large as to be completely intolerable, it is likely that public acceptance will be driven by perceived benefits. An example might be nuclear power, where very small risks to local residents may be unacceptable if the technology brings no personal benefit, but larger absolute risks (from transport hazards or medical treatment) are acceptable because of the desirability of the resulting benefits of application. It is also important to note that public perceptions change as hazards become less generic (for example, genetic modification as a science may produce very different public responses compared with specific applications of genetic modification to medicine). Michael (1992) comments that the public differentiates between science as an abstract entity (science-in-general) and as an activity directed at specific events or problems (science-in-particular). There is evidence that public attitudes and beliefs about the risks of particular technologies are crystallized by the provision of information about specific applications of these technologies, and this may reflect the lay people's preferences for information relating to concrete and tangible examples of potential technological hazards, compared with information that relates to abstract scientific principles (Frewer *et al.* 1997c).

Effective communication may change lay beliefs about a particular technological hazard if it is presented in a balanced fashion, has come from a credible source, and is honest about the particular limitations of the technology. These are also the conditions under which the beliefs of technical competence are likely to be influential (Maharik and Fischhoff 1993). People's attitudes will change if they become more knowledgable about a technology's risks and benefits, but better information may sometimes make them more favourable, and sometimes less favourable about a technology.

## Public understanding of science

Lay perceptions regarding risks are often richer and more complex than expert beliefs, involving more psychological constructs and increased multi-dimensionality (Flynn *et al.* 1993). It is now recognized that these beliefs are not irrational, but may inform the wider public debate about risk and risk management, as well as the future strategic development of the science surrounding some potential hazards (for example, in the case of emerging technologies).

In the case of different kinds of radiation hazard (including that from both natural and unnatural sources) the lay public perceives that natural sources are less threatening than artificial sources. Even for artificial sources, threat is very much related to perceptions of need or benefit. Medical radiation is much more acceptable than that associated with the nuclear industry. This may be because:

1. Artificial radiation adds risk to the environment where it was not present before. Natural radiation is tolerable as it represents part of the

natural order. The public is likely to prefer the development of alternatives to artificial radiation sources, but to be relatively indifferent in
attempting to reduce the risks from natural radiation sources.

2. There are public perceptions that the risks and benefits accruing from
   artificial radiation sources differentially affect demographic groups or
   populations. For example, the public benefits from medical radiation
   but industry benefits from nuclear power generation

Increased public understanding of science is unlikely to lead to greater
acceptance of technologies perceived as potentially risky by the public (Evans
and Durant 1995). Consider, for example, the case of genetic modification.
Effective communication of the risks and benefits of genetic modification
will not automatically lead to increased acceptance. While there has been an
historical view (from both policy-makers and scientists) that the public
should be 'educated' to accept the technology, there is evidence that increased knowledge and understanding may serve to polarize attitudes, an
effect that may be very dependent on the prior attitudes already held by the
population, as people tend to select information that is consistent with an
already held view (Frewer *et al.*, 1998*b*).

Various barriers to public understanding of science have been identified:

1. People tend to avoid learning about the underpinning science of those
   technologies which they fear, an effect similar to the 'usable ignorance'
   effect, whereby people tend to avoid information about risks associated
   with hazards to which they choose to expose themselves.

2. People express far more interest in those technologies which they believe
   are highly beneficial to society in general.

3. Public understanding of science is unlikely to have a great impact on
   public perceptions of risk unless the public also perceives that there is
   the possibility of influencing future strategic development of science.

Switzerland provides a good example of the use of referenda in the
identification and public assessment of new technologies and their future
development. Buchmann (1995) noted that the Swizz population has mixed
public opinions about new biotechnology, positive in terms of attitudes to
progress, but negative in terms of the potential for misuse, particularly
within the context of self regulation by scientists and industry. A referendum
regarding increased constitutional regulation of biotechnology was held
in 1992, which resulted in a 'yes' vote for increased regulation, which
Buchmann interpreted as indicative of a strong signal to interested institutions to consider citizens' concerns in the future development of the
technology.

# Trust in information about risk

'Who trusts whom and why' is potentially one of the most important issues in risk communication. If the government is to effectively communicate about the risks associated with different hazards, it is essential that the importance of source characteristics as potential influences on risk communication effectiveness be understood. In particular, the role of trust in information source and the impact of source credibility on reactions to risk communication may be influenced both by perceived characteristics of the hazard, and of the information source. Trusted sources (e.g. consumer organizations and medical doctors) are perceived to be both knowledgable and concerned with public welfare. Distrusted sources (e.g. the government) are perceived to distort information, to have been proven wrong in the past, and to provide biased information. Trust is associated with moderate accountability. Industry is perceived to be over-accountable, whereas the tabloid press is perceived to have too little accountability and to sensationalize risk information (Frewer *et al.* 1996).

Effective risk communication about lifestyle hazards has a different goal from that associated with technologies. In the case of behaviours which may pose direct health problems (e.g., the selection of unhealthy diets or smoking) there is no ethical problem in persuading people to change their actions in order to reduce hazard exposure, individualizing information to reduce optimistic bias effects, as well as to increase issue involvement for those most at risk. The use of persuasive information appears to increase personal risk perceptions for lifestyle hazards, which is important in terms of making the information more salient and changing behaviours (Frewer *et al.* 1997*b*). Risk information might better be provided by a highly trusted source (such as a member of the medical profession) if optimistic bias effects are to be reduced for hazards which have low personal relevance for individual members of the population (e.g. excessive alcohol use).

In the case of technological hazards, the goal of effective risk-benefit communication is to ensure that individuals make decisions about food consumption based on their knowledge of scientific assessment of risks and benefits. For example, information about genetic modification from a distrusted source appears to result in very negative attitudes if it is persuasive in content and factual presentation of both risks and benefits is important. Perceptions of trust in the information source and acceptance of emerging technologies is increased if acknowledgment is made of the uncertainties inherent in risk assessment. This implies that public understanding of the principles of scientific uncertainty is more sophisticated than assumed in the past, although clearly there is a need to investigate the impact of uncertainty on risk perceptions further (Frewer *et al.*, 1998*b*).

Finally, beliefs about risk are likely to be more difficult to change once they have been developed, as individuals tend to establish decision rules or heuristics which simplify their way of looking at the world. This is particularly true of those individuals with a low 'need for cognition', or a preference for avoiding complex and abstract thinking. Trust is likely to be a more influential cue for individuals in this group compared with those who prefer to engage in effortful processing of information. Other co-varying attitudes (e.g., concern for the environment in the case of attitudes towards emerging technologies) are good predictors of risk perceptions, although individual differences should also be taken into account. If the risk message provided opposes already established attitudes, the information source may be perceived as less credible than previously believed, which may further polarize attitudes.

It is essential to improve public trust in information sources about risk, as well as those regulatory processes that ensure public safety. This is likely to be even more important if information about risk is provided by those responsible for risk regulation. While there has been much discussion of improving transparency in the regulatory system as a means of improving consumer confidence, this may mean different things in different contexts. One context involves increased transparency in risk management processes, such that the 'weak' points in any risk assessment can be identified by other experts, and indeed the public (assuming the results of the assessment are placed in the public domain and individual members of the public have the informational 'tools' available to criticize the process). A second context involves increased transparency in terms of public scrutiny and involvement, which is dependent on effective risk communication in the first instance. Risk characterization is useful in determining public demands for risk prioritization, but it is also important to take account of public health priorities for high risk hazards which are low in terms of public priority for risk mitigation due to their voluntary nature. It is essential that expert and public models of decision-making regarding such risk mitigation priorities be developed. It is important to incorporate risk perceptions of both lay people and experts into the resulting models, and to test the actual impact these perceptions have on decision outcomes.

Another aspect of increased transparency refers to public involvement in risk-making decisions. 'Procedural justice' refers to the fairness of processes by which decisions are reached, which directly implies the need for a participatory communication process, rather than the 'top-down' approach that has been used in the past. Non-governmental organizations now have an expectation of involvement in the discussion of meaningful alternatives in the deliberation process. Such participation processes are, however, likely to fail unless the public sees the results of public involvement being incorporated into subsequent policy decisions.

## The media and risk perception

There has been much debate as to whether the media set the agenda for public debate, or merely reflect the wider public discourse about risk and associated public concerns. In very broad terms, potential media impact of this kind can be dissociated into that which is linked with risk presented in a 'crisis' context (as in the case of a 'new' hazard being suddenly identified as potentially harmful) or as a 'chronic' hazard which is constantly representative of threat. An example of 'crisis' media reporting in the UK might be the Chernobyl accident in April 1986 or the more recent BSE scare in March 1996. An example of 'chronic' risk reporting is that associated with the risks of smoking cigarettes. This is not to exclude the possibility of a chronic hazard being transformed into one associated with crisis reporting, should new scientific evidence or a change in the social context surrounding the hazard result in it being prioritized in terms of the media agenda. Likewise, a crisis could lead to a chronic aftermath.

It should also be remembered that most members of the public obtain their risk information from the media. Certain media sources have been shown to be among the most trusted sources for information about food-related risks—in particular, the quality press and television news broadcasts are highly trusted, certainly in comparison with government and industry (Frewer *et al.* 1996).

Different types of hazard are associated with very different types of risk reporting. A content analysis which examined risk reporting of different food hazards in the British quality press was conducted over a period of 1 year, from February 1992 to January 1993 (Frewer *et al.* 1993/4). The risk information associated with a range of different food hazards ('intentional food additives', 'biotechnology and genetic engineering', 'chemical and pesticide residues', 'food irradiation', 'microbiological food contamination', and 'natural toxins) was identified and quantified. It was found that the quantity of risk information associated with different hazards varied, as well as the qualitative content of the information. Microbiological hazards were associated with quantitative, statistical information. In contrast, the potential risks associated with biotechnology were presented in terms of value statements, and were linked to statements associated with the risk being unknown, and to conflict between the different 'actors' in the risk debate. To some extent this might be predicted by the nature of the hazards themselves. Finally, food additives (where a great deal of quantitative risk information was available in the scientific literature) were associated with very little risk information in the media. Rather, additives were presented as a risk, with no qualifying risk (or safety) information, thus implying that they should be avoided by the public.

Freudenberg *et al.* (1996) question whether the mass media do, in fact 'blow risks out of proportion'. The alternative argument is that the media minimize the kinds of reporting that may destabilize large-scale industries. The authors report that, in terms of actual coverage of different hazards, the most important effect in increased coverage is generated by levels of objective information, such as the numbers of casualties or the actual level of damage. However, 'keynote' effects (such as headlines and photographs), which are relatively independent of 'objective' risk information, are more important in influencing the emotional tone of the risk report—and, by implication, the risk perception of the hazard.

There is some evidence that a social amplification of risk associated with BSE occurred in the UK following the media reporting of the uncertainty surrounding the link between BSE in cattle and negative impact on human health. While the economic effects were immediate, effects on risk perception were less dramatic, although present (Fife-Schaw and Rowe 1996). The extent and content of media risk reporting about the Chernobyl accident, BSE, and some other potential hazards during the months of March, April, and May of 1996 in selected quality and tabloid newspapers in the UK were analysed. Most of the risk reporting during this period was about BSE, which first appeared in the media in a 'crisis' context in March 1996. The results of the analysis indicate that reporting of BSE increased public risk perceptions of risk associated with BSE, though this had declined by September of the same year, particularly for perceptions of personal risk. In contrast, media reporting abut the tenth anniversary of Chernobyl was reassuring, and thus served to attenuate risk perceptions. The type of newspaper was important in determining coverage of different hazards. For example, the local newspapers studied tended to be more concerned about domestic nuclear power than BSE or Chernobyl, and reporting of content reflected a local economic agenda rather than risk-related issues. It was found that the dominant national newspapers in terms of circulation, the tabloid press, used a different reporting strategy to the quality press, such that they tended to focus less on quantitative risk information. Television reporting of BSE was very similar to newspaper coverage in terms of the proportion of coverage devoted to the hazard, but contained relatively little risk information due to the brief period of time allocated. Television reporting drew the attention of the public to the risk, but did not provide detailed information about the hazard. Retrospective analysis indicated that the profile of media reporting contemporary with the Chernobyl accident had a very similar media profile to BSE ten years later, implying that media reporting of crisis may be generic and follow a natural pattern whereby the risk story is 'established' in terms of risk qualities in the first ten days after the crisis has occurred (Frewer *et al.* 1997*a*). The relatively reduced but continuous level of reporting after this date acts as a heuristic or cognitive 'trigger' which reinforces public risk perceptions created during the establishment phase. From a cognitive psychology perspective, simply but frequently repeated images are likely to result in the formation of an 'availability heuristic', or establishment of an internal rule that signifies potential danger (Tversky and Kahnemann 1984).

There is a need to further develop the social amplification of risk model in the context of risks with different psychological characteristics. This might also provide risk regulators with insights into how best to provide the media with risk information, and how to evolve an effective interface with media 'gatekeepers'.

# Future research needs

There are specific areas where further research into risk perception and risk communication is needed. In particular, little is known about the extent to which risk perception phenomena generalize across cultures. This has clear implications for understanding public responses to transboundary risks, such as genetic modification or nuclear power. It is possible that some cultures tend to make decisions based on perceptions of risk avoidance (that is, individuals have a preference for attainment of zero risk exposure) whereas others have a preference for decision-making that maximizes benefit, and risk perceptions become less important.

More research is needed in order to understand the dynamic shifts in perception and attitudes during crises. Such research must include an empirical examination of the relative importance of trust in those responsible for dealing with the risk crisis.

Appreciating the impact of source factors on the long-term effects of risk communication on attitudes and behavioural reactions is essential if the links between risk perception, risk communication, and behavioural effect are to be understood. It is also necessary to study trust in information source on reactions to information provided within a crisis context, rather than for hazards which remain relatively stable over time, particularly within the context of risk amplification and attenuation via the media. Trust and distrust in risk regulators are likely to have an influence on both risk perceptions and responses to risk communication. This is likely to be particularly important if the information source is closely associated with both the process of risk regulation and risk management.

Public understanding of the uncertainty inherent in the risk assessment process is also worthy of future research. There is extensive debate about how to increase and foster public participation in decision-making, but there is a need to understand its implications in terms of both policy formulation and resource allocation. At present, there is no cohesive and systematic understanding of the advantages and disadvantages of the different methods of providing public and stakeholder inputs into risk assessment processes, and this represents an area that is extremely important in terms of future research. Failure by risk regulators to adequately address issues of public involvement in the risk assessment process is likely to result in public perceptions that the 'real risks' are being 'hidden' because they are unacceptable to the public, further compromising trust in those responsible for risk regulation.

Other areas of social psychological theory may usefully be applied to the investigation of risk perceptions. In particular, social representation theory offers the potential to further unpack the associations between different types of hazards, as well as the strength of the psychological determinants of these risk perceptions and how these perceptions relate to behaviours and to other salient beliefs.

# Conclusions

Risk communication about different hazards is likely to be more effective it the actual concerns of the public are addressed, and these must be assessed for individual hazards. Similarly, the causes of optimistic bias or unreal optimism need to be understood within the context of particular hazards. Increased understanding of science provides the public with the ability to make informed decisions regarding risk exposure for some hazards, but does not necessarily lead to increased public acceptance of them. Other social context effects, such as trust in both information sources and risk regulators is important and must be understood in terms of effect on public risk perceptions and the development of effective communication. Future research is needed to bridge the gap between risk characterization approaches (which are descriptive, but not predictive) and risk communication models. To this end, it is also important to understand the role of the media in influencing risk perceptions, but this research must be conducted within an appropriate theoretical framework. Methods to increase public participation in risk decision-making should also be developed, in order to increase transparency in the regulatory framework as shown.

# REFERENCES

Buchmann, M. (1995). The impact of resistance to biotechnology in Switzerland: a sociological view of the recent referendum. In *Resistance to new technology*, (ed. M. Bauer, pp. 189–208. Cambridge University Press, Cambridge.

Evans, G. and Durant, J. (1995). The relationship between knowledge and attitudes in public understanding of science in Britain. *Public Understanding of Science*, **4**, 57–74.

Fife-Schaw, C. and Rowe, G. (1996). *Monitoring and modelling consumer perceptions of food-related risk.* Report to the UK Ministry of Agriculture, Fisheries and Food, London.

Fischhoff, B., Slovic, P., Lichtenstein, S., and Combs, B. (1978). How safe is safe enough? A psychometric study of attitudes towards technological risks and benefits. *Policy Studies*, **9**, 127–52.

Flynn, J., Burn,s W., Mertz, C. K., and Slovic, P. (1992). Trust as a determinant of opposition to a high level radioactive waste repository: analysis of a structural model. *Risk Analysis*, **12**, 417–31.

Flynn, J., Slovic, P., and Mertz, C. K. (1993). Decidedly different: expert and public views of risks from a radioactive waste repository. *Risk Analysis*, **13**, 643–8.

Freudenberg, W. R., Coleman, C. L., Gonzales, J., and Helgeland, C. (1996). Media coverage of hazard events—analyzing the assumptions. *Risk Analysis*, **16**, 31–42.

Frewer, L. J., Raats, M., and Shepherd, R. (1993/4). Modelling the media: the transmission of risk information in the British quality press. *Journal of the Institute of Mathematics and its Applications to Industry*, **5**, 235–47.

Frewer, L. J., Shepherd, R., and Sparks, P. (1994). The interrelationship between perceived knowledge, control and risk associated with a range of food related hazards targeted at the self, other people and society. *Journal of Food Safety*, **14**, 19–40.

Frewer, L. J., Howard, C., Hedderley, D., and Shepherd, R. (1996). What determines trust in information about food-related risks? Underlying psychological constructs. *Risk Analysis*, **16**, 473–86.

Frewer, L. J., Howard, C., Campion, E., Miles, S., and Hunt, S. (1997a). *Perceptions of radiation risk in the UK before, during and after the 10th anniversary of the Chernobyl accident.* report to the European Commission.

Frewer, L. J., Howard, C., Hedderley, D., and Shepherd, R. (1997b). The use of the elaboration likelihood model in developing effective food risk communication. *Risk Analysis*, **17**, 269–81.

Frewer, L. J., Howard, C., and Shepherd, R. (1997c). Public concerns about general and specific applications of genetic engineering: risk, benefit and ethics. *Science, Technology and Human Values*, **22**, 98–124.

Frewer, L. J., Howard, C., and Shepherd, R. (1998a). Development of a scale to assess attitudes towards technology. *Journal of Risk Research*, **1**, 221–37.

Frewer, L. J., Howard, C., and Shepherd, R. (1998*b*). The importance of initial attitudes on responses to communication about genetic engineering in food production. *Agriculture and Human Values*, **15**, 15–30.

Maharik, M. and Fischhoff, B. (1993). Risk knowledge and risk attitudes regarding nuclear energy sources in space. *Risk Analysis*, **13**, 345–53.

Michael, M. (1992). Lay discourses of science—science in general, science in particular and self. *science, Technology and Human Values*, **17**, 313–333.

Tversky, A. and Kahneman, D. (1984). Choices, values and frames. *American Psychologist*, **39**, 341–50.

Van der Pligt, J., Eiser, R., and Spears, R. (1986). Attitudes towards nuclear energy: familiarity and salience. *Environment and Behaviour*, **18**, 75–93.

Weinstein, N. D. (1980). Unrealistic optimism about future life events. *Journal of Personality and Social Psychology*, **39**, 806–20.

# 3 Public reactions to risk: social structures, images of science, and the role of trust

Ian H. Langford, Claire Marris, and Timothy O'Riordan
*Centre for Social and Economic Research on the Global Environment, School of Environmental Sciences, University of East Anglia, Norwich*

## Introduction

For 20 years, social scientists have been arguing that risk perception is a combination of culturally acquired dispositions. Within that broad phrase lie the norms of scientific analysis and peer review, expectations and doubts over 'expertise', bonding and solidarity among people that shape their views on fairness and trust, and structures of regulation that build in support or suspicion. In sum, risk perception is a collage of outlooks, predispositions, relationships, and structures all relating to each other in complex ways, like stars in a rotating galaxy.

We are at a point of ferment in the design of risk regulatory styles, organizational composition, and procedures. In the UK, the forthcoming Food Standards Agency is being shaped and designed. Its evolution, and the necessary reforms to other agencies dealing with issues such as genetically modified organisms and reportedly toxic chemicals, will map out the successes of risk perception research for the next decade. The following discussion sets the scene by considering the role of science in dealing with uncertainty. We then introduce some empirical case studies of public response to different risks, interpreting these both in terms of individual psychology and in terms of the wider social context in which individuals operate.

## Science and uncertainty

### Burdens of proof

In general, people do not want to be exposed to the possibility of risk to their health and welfare, unless they choose to be so for a perceived benefit.

Where risks are potentially widespread, long term and unavoidable, they place a great burden of proof on negative results—people want to know that something such as eating genetically modified foodstuffs is *definitely* safe. The scientific method, however, traditionally requires a greater burden of proof for positive results. Although undesirable consequences may arise from the production of false negatives, it is usually assumed that false positives pose a more inherent challenge to scientific integrity. A negative result from a study can always be accompanied by caveats about insufficient sample sizes, large standard errors, and the need for further investigation. However, a false positive may cause extensive media interest and public alarm, particularly if the research deals with a risk that attracts a fair number of 'fright factors' (see Chapter 1), with consequent costs to the public or private purse that could influence scientific reputations. As Shrader-Frechette (1996) comments:

> 'Because they are more interested in avoiding false positives (type I errors) rather than false negatives (type II errors) in situations of uncertainty, scientists place a greater burden of proof on the person who postulates some, rather than no, effect ... Although 'no effect' results run the risk of type II errors, scientists usually assume, as in criminal law, that null hypotheses are provisionally acceptable (innocent) until they are rigorously falsified (proved guilty)'.

In effect, we have a two-value frame consisting of *falsification*, where attempts are made to eliminate the likelihood of being wrong, and *provisional acceptance*, where sufficient evidence is sought to justify a particular hypothesis. However, this approach is no longer sufficient in itself to examine many risks which may be shrouded in uncertainty and coloured by political and societal contexts. Instead, judgements about risks become judgements *about the quality of the organizations and regulatory procedures* that create and monitor danger, rather than the danger itself. In this sense, therefore, risk perception is a reflection of public trust in scientific and political institutions generally. So there is much at stake.

## Science and the need for certainty

Climate change, the loss of tropical forests, endocrine-disrupting chemicals, genetically altered food products, and many other issues throw up a host of possible futures whose significance for planetary or human well-being cannot satisfactorily be analysed by scientists operating strict and two-dimensional rules. These are essentially complex and unknown phenomena, requiring the direct engagement of the public for valuation and resolution. This extended form of enquiry has been termed 'civic science' by the American environmental analyst Lee (1993). Civic science politicizes the process in the sense that science evolves via adaptive human choices about means and ends. Options for social choice are built into the prognoses: the act of creating a 'future' becomes an act of political choice that sets the conditions for shaping the next 'future'.

Procedures for deliberative, participatory, and consensus-based approaches to risk management have been examined by a number of authors. The most comprehensive studies are those by the German sociologist Renn and his colleagues (Renn *et al.* 1995) and by Irwin (1996). Both look at how trust and confidence-building come from creating respect, listening and responding, and by generating consensus out of 'side bargains'. The keys are *inclusiveness* of interested parties and *safety nets* for possible long-term liability. Inclusiveness is much more awkward to achieve than it seems, for some interests are not mobilized, and may not even know their views or positions are relevant. These are the 'fatalists' of the cultural theorists (see below), or the 'third dimension' power dependents on the famous typology of power by Lukes (1957). According to Lukes, elite interests create conditions that make the vulnerable believe that their interests are being served by being disempowered. This may be the case over consumer 'pressures' to eat clean-looking food of the same size and shape. The food may not necessarily be 'healthy' but it looks wonderful on the supermarket shelves and it is cheaper than the organic alternatives. So it becomes the 'good' food that consumers appear to want—until, that is, they hear of genetic modification.

Funtowicz and Ravetz (1996) provide an additional perspective on what they term 'post-normal' science. This applies to problems where 'facts are uncertain, values in dispute, stakes high, and decisions urgent ...'. As a result 'the typical opposition of 'hard' facts and 'soft' values is inverted; here there become decisions which are 'hard' in every sense, for which the scientific inputs are irredeemably 'soft'. This observation is not in any way an attack on science. It is simply stating that applying the rules of probability and inference to complex environmental threats provides insufficient evidence for policy makers to develop workable and socially tolerated solutions. Scientists should not disagree with this, yet scientific evidence is still seen by many, including most scientists, as somehow clean and noble, and above the mire of public debate.

## Bayesian approaches

However, changes are already occurring in the ways uncertain data are routinely analysed. Bayesian statistics are now being used to tackle a range of problems in environmental epidemiology (World Health Organisation 1999). If one takes this approach, the independence of scientific evidence is immediately seen to be untrue. Bayes' rule can be simply stated as:

prior expectation × likelihood of occurrence = posterior expectation

Hence, analysis is conditioned on the basis of prior information. One must incorporate the assumptions and expectations about outcomes before the new data are examined. If there is very limited information about a particular risk issue, one must use a very vague prior expectation. Conversely, if previous studies have already produced some firm results, such knowledge can be updated through the data currently being collected. The posterior expectation of the relationships between a potential environmental cause and a public health effect can be examined in the light of previous information and even more subjective 'expert' opinion.

To give a recent example, an article in *Nature* by Almond and Pattison (1997) on the potential links between BSE in cows and new variant Creutzfeldt-Jacob Disease (nvCJD) in humans, states, in its final paragraph:

'Finally, these latest results also do not tell us anything more about the route by which the victims of nvCJD were infected'.

Yet they then state:

'But we still think that the most likely exposure was through eating beef products that included infected offal before it was banned from human food late in 1989'.

Judgements in science, as in every other field of human activity, are based on the burden of evidence at any particular point in time. Yet it would be unwise to think that these judgements are value-free, or immune to the influences of the dominant paradigms of thought. For example, traditional epidemiology works best when there is a fairly large and specific health effect confined to a well-defined subgroup of the population and associated with a single, easily measured risk factor. Hence, epidemiologists and other researchers search for these conditions when faced with a new problem such as CJD. It is not surprising, perhaps, that the present dominant theory is of a specific disease (nvCJD) affecting a defined sector of the population (meat eaters). Almond and Pattison even speculate that the case of a vegetarian developing nvCJD may have been the result of inadvertently consumed beef products. This information is then linked to a specific risk factor, namely, consuming contaminated beef products prior to 1989. This is not to say this is mistaken, but it will be interesting to see if the final picture turns out to be more complex, e.g. requiring multiple causal agents, precursors, or particular predispositions.

What is occurring here is the complex relationship between the evolving quest for greater proof—a powerful driving force in scientific method—and the pressing need for clear judgement about policy priorities—often involving money and interest groups with political weight, and where the expectation is still to do nothing where the evidence is inconclusive. Slowly, the scientist is being tipped into the precautionary bucket, as appears to be the case with the BSE-nvCJD debate at present.

# Individual perceptions

## Trust and accountability

Studies of trust have been mentioned already in Chapters 1 and 2. A study of our own (Marris *et al.* 1996) investigated how residents of Norwich, in the East Anglian region of England, viewed trust. We found that the vast majority distinguished between the trustworthiness of sources when seeking reassurance about risks generally. Only 8% trusted the government, and, by implication, government-funded scientists. This is a somewhat worrying finding, as the huge majority of scientists working in government-funded agencies are genuinely committed to the highest codes of scientific practice. It is because their work is associated with a government ministry with 'hands in the environmental till' that the problem of trust becomes serious. Similarly only 12% trusted private companies, mostly for the same reasons. The media got little greater favour, with only 15% approval rating, while less than one-third trusted religious organizations and trades unions. Scientists associated with these institutions also become tainted.

A fairly recent MORI poll found that the proportion of the public who had either no or little confidence in scientists working for the government rose from 54% in 1993 to 62% in 1996 (Worcester 1996). Faith in scientists working for industry was greater, with only 32% expressing no, or not much, confidence. Yet this is sufficient to suggest that a company such as Shell, which successfully embarked on a £70 million public-confidence-boosting exercise over its new choice of options for the disposal of the Brent Spar oil storage platform, still faces an uphill struggle. As we shall see, any messages that Shell chooses to signal to the world ideally should vary in order to command the support of the different 'publics' who view Shell and Brent Spar so very differently.

What is noteworthy is that two major oil companies with a bad record of handling local people and indigenous cultures in their search for oil, have recently created social responsibility and ethical audits of their affairs. Shell (1998) and BP (in press) have gone on record as admitting that they had not sufficiently taken into account the social equity and care aspects of their relationships with employees, customers, and local communities. It is now high on their agenda to create a transparent and open agenda for these matters, as a trust and confidence-building exercise. This will be a long and rocky road. Because both companies have 'gone over the parapet', they will be analysed for a full account of their adventures in taking the whole social dimension seriously.

Interestingly, Peters *et al.* (1997) have found marked differences between people's expectations of different institutions within the US, namely industry, the government, and citizen groups. The government was expected to show a great deal of commitment to communicating information about environmental risks, but not to show much concern and care. In contrast, industry was expected to show concern and care when communicating risks, as well as be responsible for disclosing information. Citizen groups should have high levels of knowledge and expertise, as well as commitment. If groups do not conform to these prior expectations, they are likely to lose public trust and credibility. The scientists with the higher credibility rating in the Norwich poll received 60% support, while doctors scored 78% support. In the MORI poll, the scientists with the highest level of trustworthiness (78%) were those working for non-governmental campaigning groups or organizations (NGOs). No wonder Greenpeace moved so swiftly and comprehensively to admit its error of estimation in the toxicity of the oil-mud residues in the Brent Spar storage facility. Public trust is hard to win and easy to lose.

In the Norwich study, the somewhat surprising finding was that the two most trusted sources for people to 'hear the truth about risks' were friends (80%) and family (90%). Two implications emerge from the high ratings for NGO campaign organizations and peer-family networks. One is that the mobilized science of protest and intelligence-gathering appears to be wished for by many people who look for it to be credible. We speculate that this is because such 'popular protest' science is believed to be conducted in the public interest, and targeted against institutions that cannot be relied upon. This may explain the MORI figures and to some extent, the Norwich results. The image of science is embedded in a wider judgement of trust over the institutional setting in which the science is done. Ministry of Agriculture scientists genuinely seek to be independent, but their location in an organization perceived to be tainted by political and commercial biases swamps a view of their neutrality. That relationship should be altered with the arrival of the Food Standards Agency.

The other implication of these findings is that social bonding creates solidarities of credibility. At their core are what the UK psychologist Eiser (1994) calls 'attitudinal certainties'. People store opinions and beliefs around relatively stable self-reinforcing attitudinal structures, and seek reassurance through social bonding that is both a referent and a consequence of them.

We shall consider such social processes below. First, however, we present a model of how individuals form their perceptions of risk.

## A model for the construction of risk perceptions

An individual's perceptions of a particular risk in the environment is likely to change over time as new information is gathered. A particular attitude can be seen as having three stages: development, maintenance, and transition. Development is an interaction between external stimuli and the deeper cognitive structures already present in a person's mind. The attitude is then maintained by new information being collected, often selectively, to support it. Information may also be interpreted with bias that justifies currently held beliefs (see Chapter 1). However, new events may cause transition from one attitude or belief to another, and this change is likely to be sudden (Eiser 1994). Figure 3.1 outlines this dynamic process, the elements of which may be illustrated as follows (Langford and McDonald 1997):

1.  *Previous experiences and perceptions*: these may be accumulated factual experiences, such as 'my mother died of a brain tumour when I was a child', and include subjective interpretations of events and associations,

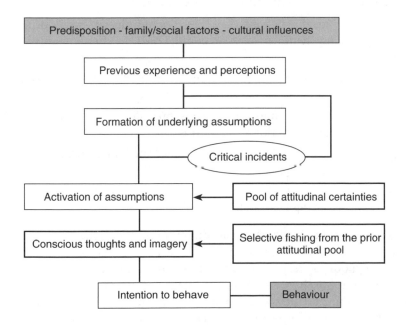

**Fig. 3.1** The dynamic nature of risk perception.

e.g. 'we lived near a chemical plant, pollution incidents were on the news a lot, but no-one did anything about it'.

2. *Formation of underlying assumptions*: these may be based on the cognitive and/or affective aspects of information processing and be represented by negative distortions, such as helplessness, e.g. 'you'll never bring anyone to account for these things—they'll always get away with it'. Conversely, positive distortions involving rationalization and denial may also play a role, e.g. 'it wouldn't happen to me. Only people who work in chemical plants are at risk, and only if they don't follow the safety precautions.' In addition, deficits in knowledge and information-processing skills may amplify these distortions, as well as an individual's ability to solve problems and come to terms with conflict.

3. *Critical incidents*: these may influence either the development or activation of underlying assumptions, e.g. 'when I heard they were planning to develop a new chemical plant near where my children live, I knew I had to do something about it myself'.

4. *Activation of assumptions*: this may be simply an accumulation of incidents leading to gradual change, but may be triggered by a specific, potentially inappropriate reaction to one incident, e.g. 'the last straw'. Changes in cognitive processing, as well as in behaviour, may well follow catastrophic or chaotic patterns (Eiser 1994).

5. *Conscious thoughts and imagery*: these may influence many aspects of life, providing reinforcement or conflict with existing cognitive structures. Effects may be:

   (1) physiological, e.g. 'I can't even get a good night's sleep worrying about it all';

   (2) cognitive, e.g. 'I find myself being preoccupied with this thing, but I think there's nothing I can do';

   (3) affective, e.g. 'I feel so anxious/frustrated/angry/depressed about this whole thing;

   (4) behavioural, e.g. 'I'm moving to a different area. I don't want my children living near a chemical plant'.

These are primarily psychosocial dimensions. We argue that any risky phenomenon fits into a collage of such beliefs. The role of the mind is to provide a 'pool' of related beliefs and attitudes into which all these new interpretations are shaped to rest. But this is not just an individual process. People are also part of social 'solidarities' through which they gain their cues for evaluating new information. This is the domain of 'cultural theory', so-called because it relies on the cultures of underlying social structures for shaping an individual's viewpoint. We respect this theory because it provides a basis for explaining why it is that public trust in handling changes seems to be so dependent on peer group support and influence.

# Setting perceptions in social context

## Cultural theory

Analysing individual perceptions can only take us so far in understanding how risk communication produces different responses in different people. We also need to look at wider societal processes, and at the nature of particular risks. In particular, Marris *et al.* (1997) found that there was far more variability around the mean level of perceived threat for some risks than others. This is partly because people do not judge riskiness on a simple linear scale, but use a number of different attributes such as voluntariness, fairness, impact on future generations, etc., as explored in 'psychometric' research (see Chapter 1 and Slovic (1992) for a fuller review). But there is more to it than that.

In the Norwich survey we also used cultural theory to provide an alternative, more sociological assessment. Cultural theory originated in the writings of the British anthropologist Mary Douglas (1970, 1982), and is well summarized by Michael Thompson *et al.* (1990). These authors believe that people form patterns of social solidarities which influence how they judge such matters as trust, fairness, blame, and accountability. These predispose people to assess the legitimacy of organizations (such as regulatory bodies) and evaluation techniques (such as eco-auditing or risk assessments) in particular ways.

Cultural theory divides society into two main dimensions. The first is the 'group' element, influencing patterns of social relationships. Some people rely on high group influence, while others do not feel the need to depend on the reference of socially respected peers. The second dimension is the 'grid' element, or the degree to which an individual's life is circumscribed by externally imposed rules or cultural expectations. For example, those who feel in a minority often seek reassurance from their fellows to maintain a legitimate identity, and will obey the norms of that minority to ensure their acceptance. Those who do not feel so circumscribed by external peer groupings will not seek the same level of conformity to establish their social identity.

Figure 3.2 portrays the typical typology of cultural theory. Fatalists may feel bonded to a larger whole, but do not operate as a distinctive group. Individualists dislike both bonding and grouping. Hierarchists accept the disadvantages of close bonding and grouping. Egalitarians seek association with each other, but reject any sense of being circumscribed by a higher social order. Thompson *et al.* (1990) have sought to show that orientations to nature also follow this typology. Fatalists see nature as a lottery, sometimes benign, sometimes malign; individualists prefer to regard nature as very resilient and robust; hierarchists recognize possible catastrophic boundaries to that resilience; while egalitarians regard nature as very vulnerable to human damage.

This division is related to an age-old distinction between patterns of informal order based on enterprise and freedom of action (individualism, or 'the market'), and the need for some kind of imposed order (or 'the hierarchy'). A third element was added, namely the sense of ethical fairness (or 'egalitarianism'), that groups apply when judging the appropriateness of market mechanisms or regulatory interventions. Completing the quadrant, the theorists identified 'fatalists', those who accepted order, but were unbonded to prevailing social patterns. Their solidarity rested on their willingness to tolerate circumstances because 'the world out there is simply too big to change'. Without the egalitarian critique, so the theory goes, markets and hierarchies both create alienated and subordinated individuals

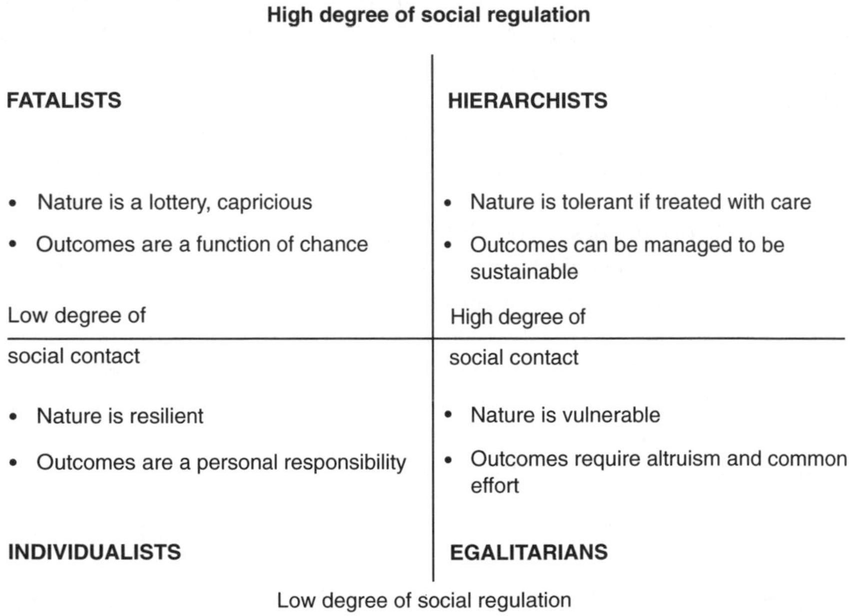

**High degree of social regulation**

| FATALISTS | HIERARCHISTS |
|---|---|
| • Nature is a lottery, capricious | • Nature is tolerant if treated with care |
| • Outcomes are a function of chance | • Outcomes can be managed to be sustainable |
| Low degree of | High degree of |
| social contact | social contact |
| • Nature is resilient | • Nature is vulnerable |
| • Outcomes are a personal responsibility | • Outcomes require altruism and common effort |
| INDIVIDUALISTS | EGALITARIANS |

Low degree of social regulation

**Fig. 3.2**   The four rationalities of human action.

(i.e. fatalists), with no solidarity except their collective sense of subordination (Thompson, personal communication).

The criticism of cultural theory comes in two forms. One is that individuals cannot be typed so easily, for they may play many roles (e.g. as a marketing manager by day and a scout leader in the evening), and organize their life in a variety of social groupings (Rayner 1992). The other critique concerns the method of assessing cultural solidarities. The charge is of reliance on psychometric techniques that merely reinforce the very patterns of attitudes being sought (Boholm 1996). By trying to ascertain a view on, say, fairness or legitimacy, the analyst assumes a predetermined set of 'rules' about fairness and legitimacy to provide the sieve for any demarcation. This is a tougher criticism to counter, but nevertheless, we found the cultural theory typology useful for calibrating different possible reactions to information about risks.

## Application to the Norwich study

As described more fully in Marris *et al.* (1996), we classified individuals according to the typology of cultural theory, and then brought together focus groups of individuals of the same predominant position to discuss a number of topics relevant to risk perception. The classification used a psychometric questionnaire developed by Dake (1991) and validated by various researchers, and respondents were also asked how they regarded various approaches to determining fairness through a series of hypothetical cases requiring an element of personal judgement. We put the two together to establish a clear grouping of 'types'. We then used these as focus groups for a series of discussions around themes assisted by the responses to risk and trust generated by the psychometric element of the questionnaire.

The focus groups revealed a remarkable homogeneity among the participants, none of whom knew each other beforehand. For example, Fig. 3.3 details the main 'majority views' of the participants with regard to a question about the acceptability of withholding knowledge from people exposed to a risk. Other strongly held views of the different groups included the following:

> *Fatalists*: risks faced in today's society were seen as part of an increasingly complex modern life, which overwhelms the ability to make sense of it. Pessimism was expressed about any beneficial changes occurring with respect to public health and other risks in present society, and participants believed that anyone could 'fiddle the statistics', and that you should trust no-one but yourself.
>
> *Hierarchists*: risks were perceived as being set in global institutional frameworks, rather than in personal lives, and people had a right to be

**Externally imposed rules**

| FATALISTS | HIERARCHISTS |
|---|---|
| • science cannot be trusted, so knowledge is never reliable | • people have a responsibility to find out the dangers they face |
| • we all opt out of society every day so we deserve to get what we avoid solving | • public protest is necessery to ensure good-quality information and sound rules |

| unbonded | bonded |
|---|---|
| • people should trust themselves to get informed on personal (inner) risk | • governments and corporations cannot be trusted to inform because they are fuelled by vested interests |
| • people should find out whom to trust regarding quality knowledge for societal (outer) risks | • knowledge is corrupted even when it is made available |

| INDIVIDUALISTS | EGALITARIANS |
|---|---|

**Internally imposed rules**

**Fig. 3.3**  Responses to key statement: 'A risk is less acceptable if knowledge is withheld from the people who are exposed to it'.

informed by reliable sources giving the best information about the risks in their lives. Honest reporting, trial and error, and knowledge gained by experience were seen as essential characteristics of good risk communication.

*Individualists*: the emphasis for this outlook is on personal responsibility, towards the gathering of correct information, and maintenance of social networks that can provide this. Responsibility is devolved to an individual level, where others can be activated into collective action, but collective mechanisms of operation are not maintained for their own sake.

*Egalitarians*: risks are perceived as being embedded within a much deeper set of social anxieties, and the current mode of risk management and communication in society is seen as inflaming rather then dispersing these anxieties. Only structural change in society can bring about change in the ways risks are dealt with, and the evolution of democratic processes and public participation was seen as part of this change.

## Some conclusions

This analysis suggests that no particular form of risk communication is likely to please everyone. Nevertheless, the following case studies show that some common ground may be found in the way risks are managed. For the present, we note that perception of risk is located in two sets of psychosocial processes.

> *As individuals*, we look for pools of supportive attitudinal perceptions when responding to information, or communication, about risks. These pools are generally stable, but may 'pour' into other pools if events trigger some sort of 'convulsive' reinterpretation. This took place for many in the early days of the BSE crisis and, we believe, is now occurring for many in the light of the genetically modified organism (GMO) controversy.

> *As cultural types,* we develop outlooks on the world, set more or less in response to our social groupings and external influences, that provide us with a set of judgements about the fairness and reliability of communication about risk, and how that should be handled in the form of trustworthiness.

Put these two together, and there is a complex, but predictable, basis for developing communication in setting up risk-regulatory institutions. We return to this below. Meanwhile, we provide two more pieces of casework to show how risk communication operates.

# Further studies

## Case study 2: Willingness to pay for clean bathing water

In the summers of 1995 and 1997, two surveys were undertaken to establish whether holiday-makers, day-trippers, and locals at the seaside resorts of Great Yarmouth and Lowestoft in eastern England were willing to pay higher water rates (charges) for less polluted bathing water (Georgiou *et al.* 1998). Focus groups were also used to discuss some important issues in more depth, broadly following the methodology deployed in the first case study.

From an individual psychometric view, using the cognitive model portrayed in Fig. 3.1 uncovered significant differences in perception between the two sites. At the time of the survey Lowestoft had passed the EC Bathing Water Directive Standard and Great Yarmouth had failed. The particular Directive lays down indicators of bathing water quality before any beach can be certified as 'blue' or 'safe'. At Lowestoft, 61% of the sample were aware of Lowestoft's 'clean beach' status, although there were differences between subgroups, with 71% of local residents, 65% of day-trippers, and 46% of holiday-makers having this knowledge. In other words, visitors and locals were well informed. In addition, visitors with a previous experience of illness (personally or in their family), which they attributed to bathing in polluted waters, were selecting Lowestoft as it had a 'clean beach'. In terms of Fig. 3.1, previous negative experience had prompted them to seek information and change their behaviour to visit cleaner beaches. Further, those who bathed in the sea were willing to pay significantly larger amounts to maintain the good quality of bathing water. Hence, people appeared to be behaving rationally, and the EC Directive, seen in the context of delivering a public health message, was working well in delivering that message .

At Great Yarmouth a very different picture emerged. Only 12% of the whole sample knew that the beach had failed the EC standard. Although 50% of locals were aware of this fact, only 9% of day-trippers and 7% of holiday-makers were. Furthermore, visitors to Great Yarmouth not only showed a much lower interest in bathing water quality, but those who actually bathed had a significantly *lower* willingness to pay for improved quality than those who did not. Subsequent analysis suggested that bathers at Great Yarmouth were denying there was a possible health threat, and just wanted to get on with their holiday.

The lesson here is that risk communication about public health tends to work *selectively*, and often reaches those who are *already* better informed. Interestingly, in the focus groups, there was a consensus for the provision of continuous monitoring, where information on water quality is clearly sign-posted at regular intervals, rather than adherence to some arbitrary fixed standard that is updated less often. This approach is already being implemented at some beaches in Norfolk.

As far as willingness to pay for improvements was concerned, residents at Great Yarmouth, aware of the continuing poor quality of water, seemed fed up and felt they should not be forced to pay any more. They had lost their trust in regulatory agencies and saw themselves as *victims requiring compensation*. This was not the case at Lowestoft, where residents were willing to pay for more. Overall, over 40% of respondents refused to pay anything more in water rates, despite stating that this was an important issue. The main two reasons given were distrust of government (this was prior to the May 1997 election) and outrage at the salaries being paid to water company directors. In addition, hierarchists and individualists were both more likely to accept the use of willingness to pay methods to tackle environmental health problems. Egalitarians were more likely to protest against the use of economic valuation. Fatalists would protest due to lack of trust in the relevant institutions and lack of belief that anything would be done.

This study also shows that perceptions of risk relate, in part, to judgements about the institutions creating and regulating the risk. Thus government was distrusted by almost all respondents, even hierarchists. The water companies were seen as project mongers, not particularly interested in the public good. Their public relations image was poor, and the communication strategies which they used tended to alienate, especially the egalitarians. Thus, risk management becomes a 'whole management issue' and not just for a particular section of business.

## Gender differences in perception of risk of malignant melanoma

Students at University College, Suffolk were asked about their knowledge and attitudes to the risk of malignant melanoma skin cancer from exposure to sunlight. In addition, they were asked to detail their past experiences of being sunburned, and their current behaviour regarding sunbathing and use of sunscreens. We found interesting gender differences which may explain why more women in the UK get malignant melanoma, but more men die from it (Langford et al. in press).

Young women (16–19 year olds) were significantly more likely to be aware of the risks of malignant melanoma than their male counterparts (79% compared to 34%). Most gathered their information not from health promotion material (29%), but from the mass media such as television (51%) and magazines (40%). Females were significantly more likely to use protection against the sun, such as sunscreens, and to apply it correctly and regularly. Despite this, however, females were also more likely to sunbathe to get a suntan. This seems irrational, but we also asked some questions about their opinions about themselves. Females were significantly more likely to feel unhappy if their friends had a suntan and they did not. This could be seen as a simple case of media manipulation of young women, but then males were significantly more likely to state that 'pale people are not pretty'. Therefore, in order to increase their chances of getting a partner, females were rationally choosing to take the health risk of getting a suntan, relying on the protective factors of sunblocks and timing of exposure. Remember, this is a case of socially mediated voluntary exposure, so the communication issue is more one of information, advice, and the slow shift of cultural norms towards suntan, rather than the more complex trust-related communications for involuntary exposure. Again, providing a public health message in the sunbathing context is a complex issue, requiring genuine changes in the opinions and behaviour of both sexes. Of interest here is the finding that females were more likely to go to the doctor, and be interested in their health. So, if they did develop a possible melanoma they would be more likely to seek advice and treatment. Early detection is linked to survival from the disease.

# Conclusions and discussion

## General

Public reactions to risk are very varied, according both to personal histories and outlooks, and to the influences of social bonding. Both intertwine to produce diverse, but predictable, interpretations of both voluntary and imposed dangers. From the point of view of risk communication, the key messages are:

- to be inclusive of all points of view and social networks
- to grant respect and responsiveness to all interested parties involved in discussions and debate
- to ensure that there is a 'safety net' of protection, should reasonable safety procedures be found inadequate at a later date, and to indicate beforehand how such arrangements will be put in place and be made accessible
- to recognize that certain groups in society need different forms of message about trust, liability, fairness, and accountability
- to bear in mind that risk perceptions can only finally be set in a more participatory science and democracy, and act accordingly to make both of these processes more transparent and accessible.

## Trust and accountability

These are key themes in getting people to listen, change their attitudes, and eventually change their behaviour. In the absence of trust, some health messages may be ignored, while other issues are blown out of all proportion. Independent regulatory agencies (such as the forthcoming Food Standards Agency), accountable to but independent of government, are required to provide a backdrop of reliable information for the public. The bathing water quality study showed how people will distance themselves from the process of public health management when the regulators are perceived as untrustworthy and uncaring. Even given public trust, translating health information into health action is not an easy target, as most people form habits which are hard to change, stick with the familiar, and take the route of least resistance. There may also be good reasons, in the short term, for taking some risks for perceived social benefits, as shown in the sunbathing example.

The implications for the style of regulation and communication, as well as for the structure of bodies such as the new Food Standards Agency, are that:

(1) the agency must unequivocally be seen to be independent of government, the food industry, and leading consumer and environmental groups;

(2) the Board will nevertheless need to include representatives of all these groups, with a bias towards consumer groups and independently funded scientists;

(3) the minutes of the Board should be on the Internet, with a facility for open dialogue on the web between interested parties and the Agency's policy arm;

(4) contentious issues such as that of GMOs in foods should be brought fully into the remit of the Agency;

(5) working groups on particular topics, including communication, issues management, public relations, and educational responsibilities, will require inclusive stakeholder representation and full transparency;

(6) the handling of the early decisions on food safety will set the marker for public trust.

All this may look very didactic and formidable. However, good Internet organization, well chosen Board and working group membership, an efficiently run network of communication, and clear, thoughtful, early decisions will enable this Agency to get on with its job with cooperative stakeholder relationships from its very start.

## REFERENCES

Almond, J. and Pattison, J. (1997). Human BSE. *Nature*, **389**, 437–8.

BP. (1999). Health, Safety and Environmental Reports. Internet www.bpamoco.com.

Boholm, A. (1996). Risk perception and social anthropology: critique of cultural theory. *Ethos*, **61**, 64–84.

Dake, C. (1991). Orienting dispositions in the perception of risk: an analysis of contemporary world views and cultural biases. *Journal of Cross-Cultural Psychology*, **23**, 61–82.

Douglas, M. (1970). *Cultural bias*. Occasional paper No.35. Royal Anthropological Institute, London. Republished in Douglas, M. (1982). *The active voice*, pp. 183–254. Routledge and Kegan Paul, London.

Eiser, R. (1994). *Attitudes, chaos and the connectivist mind*. University of Exeter Press, Exeter.

Funtowicz, S. O. and Ravetz, J. R. (1996). Risk management, post normal science, and extended peer communities. In *Accident and design: contemporary debates in risk* management, (ed. D. C. K. Jones and C. Hood), pp. 172–81. UCL Press, London.

Georgiou, S., Langford, I. H., Bateman, I. J., and Turner, R. K. (1998). Determinants of individuals willingness to pay for reductions in environmental health risks: a case study of bathing water quality. *Environment and Planning A*, **30**, 577–94.

Lee, K. (1993). *Compass and gyroscope: integrating science and policy for the environment*. Island Press, New York.

Irwin, A. (1996). *Citizen science*. Routledge, London.

Langford, I. H. and McDonald, A-L. (1997). *Risk perception, health and environmental change: a multidimensional model*. CSERGE Working Paper GEC 97–14, School of Environmental Sciences, University of East Anglia, Norwich.

Langford, I. H., Moulden-Horrocks, S., Day, R., McDonald, A-L., Bateman I. J., and Saunders, C. (1998). Perceptions of risk of malignant melanoma skin cancer from sunlight: a comparative study of young people in the UK and New Zealand. *Risk, Decision and Policy*, **33**, 1–12.

Lukes, S. (1957). *Power: a radical view*. Macmillan, Basingstoke.

Marris, C., Langford, I., and O'Riordan, T. (1996). *Integrating sociological and psychological approaches to public perceptions of environmental risks: detailed results from a questionnaire survey*. CSERGE Working Paper GEC 96–07, School of Environmental Sciences, University of East Anglia, Norwich.

Marris, C., Langford, I., and O'Riordan, T. (1997) Exploring the psychometric paradigm: comparisons between aggregate and individual analyses. *Risk Analysis*, **17**, 303–12.

Peters, R. G., Covello, V. T., and McCallum, D. B. (1997). The determinants of trust and credibility in environmental risk communication: an empirical study. *Risk Analysis*, **17**, 43–54.

Rayner, S. (1992). Cultural theory and risk analysis. In *Social theories of risk*. (ed. S. Krimsky and D. Golding), pp. 83–115. Praeger, New York.

Renn, O., Webber, T. O., and Wiedermann, P. (ed.) (1995). *Fairness and competence in citizen participation: evaluating models and environmental discourse*. Kluwer, Dorderecht.

Shrader-Frechette, K. (1996). Methodological rules for four classes of scientific uncertainty. In *Scientific uncertainty and environmental problem solving*, (ed. J. Lemons), pp. 12–39. Blackwell, Oxford.

Shell Oil Company (1998). *Social responsibilities report*. Internet: www.shell.com.

Slovic, P. (1992). Perception of risk: reflections on the psychometric paradigm. In *Social theories of risk,* (ed. S. Krimsky and D. Golding ), pp. 84–116. Praeger, New York.

Thompson, M., Ellis, R., and Wildavsky, A. (1990). *Cultural theory*. Westview Press, Boulder Colo.

World Health Organisation (1999). *Disease mapping and risk assessment*. Policy document, in press.

Worcester, R. (1996). *Greening the millennium: public opinion and the environment*. MORI, London.

# 4 Public and professional perceptions of environmental and health risks

Emma Green, Simon D. Short, Raquel Duarte-Davidson, and Leonard S. Levy
*MRC Institute for Environment and Health, University of Leicester*

## Introduction

Society has become increasingly conscious of its vulnerability to environmental and health risks, and recent experiences such as the bovine spongiform encephalopathy (BSE) crisis have led to a decline in confidence in the systems designed to safeguard the health and well-being of the population. Recently efforts have been directed towards improving the credibility of, and confidence in, these systems across a broad range of risk issues in public policy. It is now well established that risk judgements can vary considerably between expert and lay populations. Research on the perception of risk attributes this variance to the different understanding of risk, above and beyond statistical probability estimates, which lay people apply when making judgements about risks and their acceptability.

Qualitative hazard characteristics, along with a range of psychosocial and cultural factors, shape individual and social responses to risk (Royal Society 1992; Adams 1995). Questions of trust and credibility, particularly in relation to the institutions charged with determining acceptable levels and with the management and communication of risk, also appear to be of particular importance (Renn and Levine 1991; Slovic 1993; Marris *et al.* 1996). It is believed that the accuracy of knowledge about a hazard is potentially important in influencing the perception of risk (Bostrom *et al.* 1992). For example, it has been demonstrated that expert judgements can be prone to the same biases as those of the lay person, particularly when forced to go beyond the limits of available data and rely on intuition (Slovic 1987). In addition, research suggests that the context in which risk judgements are made, notably occupational and non-occupational settings, can influence responses to risk (Ferguson *et al.* 1994). While a number of studies have been undertaken to explore the influence of media coverage, the role of the media in generating individual perceptions and social responses to risk remains uncertain (Combs and Slovic 1979; Frewer *et al.* 1993; Freudenburg *et al.* 1996).

Considering the complexity of factors that influence responses to risk, it has become clear that communication about environmental and health risks aimed simply at the provision of quantitative information alone is likely to be of limited value. Instead, communication is more effective in achieving its goals if it is sensitive to the broad concept of risk. The effectiveness of risk messages will, therefore, be increased if they aim to address, or at least recognize, the underlying qualitative dimensions (e.g. individual risk perceptions, cultural values, and questions of trust) that shape the perception of risk. This paper discusses implications of a recently conducted pilot study into public and professional concerns about environmental and health risks. Selected results are used to illustrate some key factors which influence responses to risk, and implications for risk communication in public health are discussed.

## Some key concepts concerning the perception of environmental health risks

Any sensible discussion of risk perception and communication involves identifying which issues worry, or do not worry, individuals or groups, and why people hold a particular view. Selected environmental and health issues are explored here to illustrate key risk perception themes, and to provide some ideas as to why particular issues provoke high levels of concern while others are virtually ignored. It is one of the continuing fallacies of risk perception and communication that information necessarily equates to understanding. While it is commonly held that the public's reaction to certain risk issues is based on a misunderstanding of the information behind that issue, the large body of research on risk perception has shown that it is less a case of misunderstanding, as of understanding and reacting to information in a different, but no less valid, way.

Much of the early work on risk perception and risk communication stemmed from psychological studies on individuals' responses to a range of hazards. From this work, certain characteristics or 'fright factors' have been identified that are important in shaping perceptions. In a recent government publication, the most notable fright factors that tend to make public health risks more worrying, or less acceptable, were described (Box 1.1; Department of Health 1997). Other approaches to risk perception have explored the cultural dimensions that shape individual and group responses to risk. This research has shown that the beliefs, attitudes, and behaviour that make individuals part of a social group can also affect their perception of risks.

## Assessing public and professional concern about environmental health issues

This paper discusses selected findings of a pilot study designed to assess concern about environmental and health issues from both public and professional perspectives. The study aimed to elicit issues of concern from professionals actively involved in the management and communication of environmental and health risks, namely Environmental Health Officers (EHOs) and Directors of Public Health (DsPH). Issues of concern to the public as perceived by those professionals were also investigated. In the UK EHOs undertake administration, inspection, education, and regulation responsibilities in relation to environmental health. Environmental Health Officers are principally employed by local authorities, although an increasing number are employed by central government and industry. Within the public service an EHO has the following functions (Department of Environment/Department of Health 1996):

(1) to improve human health and protect it from environmental hazards;

(2) to maintain public health, including the control of communicable diseases, food poisoning, and infestation;

(3) to enforce environmental legislation;

(4) to develop liaison between local communities, the local authority, and between the local and higher levels of administration;

(5) to provide independent and expert advice on environmental matters; and

(6) to implement health education programmes to promote an understanding of environmental principles.

Within the National Health Service (NHS), departments of public health ensure that public health considerations, including environmental factors, are taken into account in the promotion and delivery of health care. A Director of Public Health (DPH), therefore, plays a strategic role in the promotion of public health to ensure that local authority and health authority plans and services are consistent, comprehensive, and complementary. The responsibilities of a DPH may include (Department of Environment/Department of Health 1996):

(1) the provision of public health input to the development of central policy and strategy development;

(2) the delivery of national public health support functions such as cancer registries;

(3) the provision of support for NHS activity in the control of communicable disease and non-communicable environmental exposures;

(4) the implementation of public health policy initiatives such as the *Our Healthier Nation Strategy* (UK Government 1998);

(5) the assessment of local health needs and the implementation of local health promotion strategies;

(6) the development of relationships between health authorities, clinicians, local authorities, and the local communities;

(7) the surveillance, monitoring, and control of communicable disease and environmental exposures; and

(8) the provision of a focal point for public health advice and information.

The study described here was based on a postal questionnaire survey of EHOs and DsPH in Great Britain. The objective was to identify risk issues and specific compounds that cause concern to the general population and to practitioners in the field of environmental health as a result of their professional activities. While the questionnaire aimed to identify issues of concern to the public, results from the study do not provide a direct measure of public concern (as they do for professional concern), but rather indicate likely concerns as perceived by professionals in the field (notes to the questionnaire specified that 'public concern may be indicated by issues which generate a significant number of enquiries, complaints, or requests for advice or assistance'). Following preliminary research that encompassed a broad range of organizations, a number of environmental and health issues and specific compounds were selected for inclusion as questionnaire items. The questionnaire was circulated to 114 EHOs and 120 DsPH across Great Britain and a combined response rate of 74% was achieved. The EHO sample was based on a judgement sampling procedure: Chief Environmental Health Officers were selected by administrative region with at least two councils selected for each region. These included county councils, metropolitan councils, district councils, and unitary councils and covered areas ranging from those dominated by heavy industry and urbanization to rural and sparsely populated ones. For the DsPH survey, all Health Authorities across Great Britain were contacted.

It is important that the limitations of the study are recognized. First, the questionnaire may have acted to 'bring to mind' those items presented, while omitting ones that might be of equal, or possibly greater, concern (although respondents were invited to add additional items which they considered to be of importance). Secondly, as with all research of this kind, question form and wording may play a role in the shaping of responses. While efforts were made in the wording of questions to minimize variation in the basis upon which respondents rated concern, some respondents may have indicated high levels of concern for issues which take up a lot of their time, while others rated items which they believed to be a health concern of importance.

## Understanding concerns about environmental and health issues

Results discussed below focus on environmental and health issues of concern rather than on specific compounds. From the survey of EHOs, the issues about which they were most concerned, and about which they thought the public were most concerned, were noise pollution and outdoor air quality. For DsPH, outdoor air quality and industrial waste disposal were the issues of most concern from a professional perspective, while BSE and outdoor air quality rated as issues of most concern from a public perspective ('most concern' reflects a combination of responses in the 'very concerned' and 'quite concerned' categories of the questionnaire). Table 4.1 lists the issues included in the questionnaire and shows which ones were perceived as being of greatest concern. Figure 4.1 illustrates some of these issues (bold in Table 4.1) and highlights similarities and differences between public and professional perspectives. These are discussed in detail below.

The risk associated with BSE has been in the news for over a decade and provides a classic example of a '*dread*' risk. This dread stems from the certainty that the disease is fatal and involves a particularly unpleasant death. As illustrated in Table 4.1 and Fig. 4.1 there is a high degree of consistency across professional and public perspectives for levels of concern about the risk associated with BSE. Many factors interact to make BSE such a concern. Not only is it perceived to be little understood by the scientific community, but it is also an unfamiliar disease and very few people have direct experience of it. The risk can also be described as being involuntarily imposed (initially at least, it was considered to be out of the individual's control) and recent attention has focused on the possibility of large-scale exposure with the long-term potential to affect many thousands of individuals. In reality, around 35 cases of new variant Creutzfeld Jacob Disease (nv CJD) have been confirmed (up to early 1999) and yet many hundreds of thousands of people probably ate beef in the last decade. Even if only a small

**Table 4.1**  Environmental and health issues of concern—overall rank of each item as an issue of concern from professional and public perspectives[a]

| Issue | EHOs | DsPH | EHOs (public) | DPHs (public) |
|---|---|---|---|---|
| **Outdoor air quality**[b] | 2 | 1 | 2 | 2 |
| **BSE**[b] | 4 | 4 | 3 | 1 |
| **Noise pollution**[b] | 1 | 10 | 1 | 7 |
| Drinking water quality | 9 | 6 | 4 | 3 |
| Emissions from incinerators (PCBs and dioxins) | 4 | 9 | 5 | 4 |
| Polluted lakes, rivers, and seas | 6 | 5 | 6 | 6 |
| Disposal of industrial waste | 9 | 2 | 7 | 5 |
| Poor housing and diet | 3 | 3 | 9 | 11 |
| Use of pesticides | 8 | 7 | 8 | 8 |
| Radioactive waste | 15 | 12 | 10 | 8 |
| **Indoor air quality**[b] | 5 | 7 | 16 | 17 |
| Disposal of household waste | 11 | 11 | 11 | 14 |
| Pesticide residues in food | 12 | 13 | 14 | 10 |
| Lead in drinking water | 13 | 13 | 13 | 12 |
| Genetically modified organisms | 17 | 16 | 15 | 13 |
| Use of nitrates and phosphates | 16 | 15 | 17 | 15 |
| Chlorine-based chemicals | 14 | 17 | 17 | 16 |
| Light pollution | 19 | 19 | 12 | 19 |
| Environmental oestrogens | 18 | 18 | 19 | 18 |

[a] The ranking of each item relates to the number of respondents who scored each issue as one of high concern. In this table the issue of highest concern is indicated as having a rank of 1 and the issue of least concern a rank of 19.
[b] See Fig. 4.1.

percentage of these people contract nv CJD, the perception is that many more cases must appear.

The role of the media in generating and directing public responses to risks is somewhat unclear, and this has been illustrated by the BSE crisis. While heavy media coverage appears to stimulate social responses to risk, it does not necessarily result in heightened individual concern. The important issue is how an event is processed by the media and interacting social groups (Kasperson et al. 1988; Weigman and Gutterling 1995).

Clearly the controversy surrounding BSE was influenced by uncertainty and disagreement among the scientific community and regulators. Throughout the crisis messages from the Government and other bodies designed to reassure individuals about the risks associated with BSE fuelled the controversy because they were contradictory and judged to be inconsistent with previous messages and policies. Within this framework, issues of trust became increasingly important, and confidence in risk management institutions was diminished. The experience of the BSE crisis, therefore, illustrates how the perception of and social response to risk

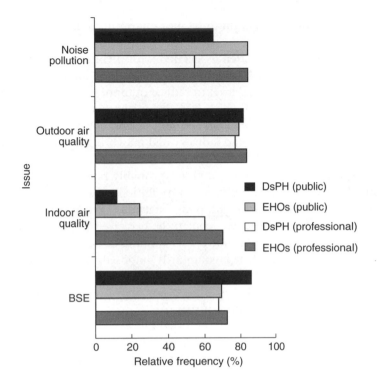

**Fig. 4.1** Levels of concern about selected environmental and health issues from public and professional perspectives.

are greatly influenced by trust in government, industry, and science as a whole.

In contrast to the consistent pattern of concern associated with BSE (Fig. 4.1), a notable difference between professional and public perspectives was recorded for indoor air quality. This difference is particularly marked when compared with the consistently high levels of concern for outdoor air quality. Concern about outdoor air quality has been identified in other surveys. For example, a 1993 survey of England and Wales which examined concerns, attitudes, and behaviour in relation to the environment found that 40% of respondents expressed high levels of concern about traffic exhaust fumes and urban smog (Department of Environment 1994). As in the pilot study described here, differences in levels of concern for outdoor air quality and indoor air quality from a public perspective have been recorded in a study on air pollution, health, and asthma (Health Education Authority/ Institute for Environment and Health 1997). In this study more people considered outdoor air pollution to be more harmful to health than indoor air pollution.

Outdoor air pollution is often associated with involuntary exposure and lack of control over the risk (although in reality there are measures which may be taken at an individual level to reduce outdoor air pollution, such as avoiding unnecessary car journeys). It is also likely that the management of risks associated with outdoor air pollution are considered to be the responsibility of government and industry and may bring into play questions of trust and credibility. These factors tend to result in heightened anxiety or a low level of risk acceptance, and are probably reinforced by the large amount of media coverage outdoor air pollution receives, thereby maintaining it as an issue high on the public agenda. In contrast, indoor air pollution, from a lay perspective, tends to be perceived as posing a low risk to health because it occurs in one's own home and is, therefore, believed to be controllable rather than involuntarily imposed. It is also likely that indoor air pollution is less frequently related to industry and, therefore, is not the blame or responsibility of others, nor does it raise questions about equity and the social distribution of risk.

In relation to noise pollution, EHOs rated this as the most important issue of concern to them and the public. In contrast, DsPH ranked it only tenth from their viewpoint and seventh from the public's viewpoint. This disparity between the attitudes of DsPH and EHOs is probably related to their different professional remits. Neighbourhood noise is a particular concern causing considerable stress and other health effects, with complaints to local authorities rising steeply. As practitioners who have daily contact with the communities they serve, EHOs probably deal more frequently with nuisance from noise than do DsPH; this highlights the possible role of the 'availability heuristic' (a risk is judged to be probable or frequent when it can easily be brought to mind). What is it about noise that makes it such a concern, especially for EHOs and the public? Noise is very close in space and time, and is involuntarily imposed on individuals who have very little control over their exposure. Environmental noise, caused by traffic, industrial, and recreational activities is an important local environmental problem in Europe, and the source of an increasing number of complaints from the public (Commission of the European Communities 1996). It has long been recognized that high levels of noise can have detrimental effects on hearing, and evidence exists to suggest that environmental noise is also linked to other health effects such as annoyance, sleep disturbance, and even ischaemic heart disease (Institute for Environment and Health 1997). For these reasons noise pollution has been identified as a target issue to be addressed under the UK's National Environmental Health Action Plan (Department of the Environment/Department of Health 1996).

# Discussion

## Implications for risk communication in public health

A large body of research shows that people (particularly when asked about risks outside their area of expertise) apply a complex understanding of risk when making personal judgements about risks and their acceptability. It has become clear that communication about environmental and health risks aimed at the provision of quantitative information alone is likely to be of limited value. Instead, communication which is sensitive to the broad concept of risk is more likely to achieve its aims.

Concentrating on the provision of opportunities for individuals to make informed decisions about whether or not to accept a particular risk, or to take certain risk-reducing actions, the discussion above draws out some important considerations for risk communication. Communication can serve a number of purposes ranging from the development of risk management policies to informing people about the various risks to which they are exposed and includes:

(1) statutory requirements to inform the public and other bodies about certain large-scale technological risks;

(2) communication of technical information between scientists, policy-makers, and risk managers to inform decision-making;

(3) communication between all stakeholder groups to inform decision-making (stakeholders are those individuals and parties concerned with, or affected by, a risk management problem and may include public interest groups, scientists, policy-makers, and risk managers); and

(4) provision of information which allows individuals to make informed decisions about whether to accept a risk or not, and to take certain risk-reducing actions.

Using information about the qualitative dimensions of risk is, therefore, important for communicating about risk as well as for the development of policies aimed at protecting public health. It can make a valuable contribution towards the implementation of effective, relevant, and meaningful communication between practitioners charged with communicating about risks and implementing risk management policies, and the communities they work with. By understanding why a particular view or concern is held, opportunities to gear information to the needs, values, and perceptions of the intended audience can be increased, and uptake of that information encouraged. Uptake of information can also be improved by exploring the preferred forms of delivery for different risk messages. In short, by endeavouring to address, or at least recognize, the broad concept of risk, the provision of information and advice about environmental and health risks can be better targeted, thus promoting take-up by intended audiences.

The inclusion of an evaluation process in communication is an important, if somewhat neglected, issue. Evaluation provides a tool by which the uptake of information or advice can be assessed, including whether information is translated into behavioural changes consistent with risk reduction, or other desired outcomes. By evaluating risk communication, more effective processes or alternative forms of information delivery and information content may be identified. This would be of particular value in circumstances where scientific knowledge about the risk advances, or where understanding of the sociopolitical context of the risk changes. For example, failure of risk information to achieve its goals may stem from gaps in understanding the relationship between individual perceptions and behaviour, and wider cultural and institutional considerations, as illustrated by the BSE crisis. On the other hand, understanding the contextual nature of risk can greatly enhance the success of risk communication. For example, a preventive policy involving the provision of health education and voluntary testing advocated consistently across government, medical, and citizen bodies has proved successful in the management of the risks associated with HIV and AIDS in the UK. While gaps in scientific knowledge existed, an understanding of the relationship between certain behaviours and the extent of infection among specific populations led to a clearer understanding of the disease. This made for greater precision in the quality of information available and the ways in which it was distributed (Scott and Freeman 1995).

## Implications for participatory approaches in decision-making

Information about the qualitative dimensions of risk can also help to inform the development and implementation of policies and decisions aimed at protecting public health. While the development of opportunities for public participation in public health is a complex and variable process, overall experience suggests that policies and decisions made in collaboration with stakeholders tend to be more effective and durable.

The management of environmental and health risks is increasingly being implemented outside traditional government arenas, for example, by industry, workers, individuals, and advocacy groups. This changing environment has led to calls for a greater involvement of those affected by risk problems in the decision-making process. A good risk management decision possesses a number of dimensions which are best identified by endeavouring to ensure stakeholder input during the decision-making process. While such decisions may primarily be based on the best scientific and technical information available, their success is also dependent on sensitivity to a range of social, economic, legal, and political considerations.

Public health policy is the process by which society collectively assures conditions in which people can be healthy. Therefore, risk management processes for public health should reflect the values of the many publics to which they are directed. The challenge for all those involved in the field is to explore possibilities for engaging relevant stakeholders throughout the process (Fig. 4.2), while ensuring that the nature and extent of participation is reflected by the scope and impact of the particular risk problem in question. Again, this requires effective communication, underpinned by an appreciation of the many different views and values held between all parties involved.

## Implications for future research

Along with an appreciation of the factors that influence responses to risk and the efficacy of information and advice, the formulation of effective risk messages is also dependent on determining the accuracy of knowledge about the risk in question, and on identifying preferred sources and forms of information regarding the risk. The study described above forms part of an ongoing research programme aimed at improving our understanding of risk perception and communication in relation to risks to health from routine levels of exposure to environmental pollutants. Results from the study have been used to select a small number of environmental and health

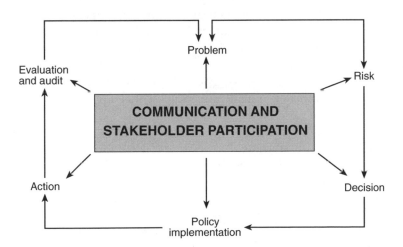

**Fig. 4.2**  Opportunities for participation in public health.

issues that warrant further attention under this programme. For example, a larger scale, public-orientated survey aimed at establishing levels of awareness, concern, knowledge, and information preferences has recently been conducted in relation to indoor air quality. This ongoing research will help to inform the formulation of relevant and targeted information material. In the wider context, the value of generic criteria for effective risk communication (applicable to a broad spectrum of environmental and health risks) will be explored.

Through a proactive approach this study has helped to narrow down key issues that warrant attention, thereby making effective use of limited resources. However, the picture presented is a 'snap-shot' of concerns at the time of the study. Because environmental and health concerns are likely to change for a variety of reasons, it would be informative to conduct longitudinal studies, or at least a series of cross-sectional studies, over time. The study benefited by drawing on the experience of practitioners who are responsible for implementing risk management policies and information programmes. These professionals often represent early points of contact for the communities they serve and, therefore, play a potentially valuable 'gate-keeper' role. However, particular care must be taken to avoid the over-interpretation of results and it should be borne in mind that the study only provided a 'surrogate' measure of public concern. An investigation among a representative sample of the population would be of value in determining the validity of, and potential for, using surrogate measures of public concern in future work.

In relation to the management and communication of public health risks there are clearly many other areas which warrant further study in order to increase the efficacy of communication and encourage a greater degree of public participation in decision-making. In particular, while the role of the media in generating individual and social responses to risk remains uncertain, it clearly constitutes a significant source of the public's information about a wide range of risk issues. Further examination of this issue could lead to a valuable insight into the potential for the media to play a positive role in risk communication. The relationships between risk perception, communication, and behavioural responses at both individual and social levels also warrants further study. The 'social amplification of risk' framework provides a useful tool for integrating apparently competing perspectives in this field, and through its application to empirical data there is a possibility that the interrelationships between perception, communication, and response may be unravelled. This type of research could provide policy- and practitioner-relevant outputs to inform efforts aimed at increasing public participation and formulating successful risk communication.

# Conclusions

Effective communication plays a vital role in the maintenance and improvement of public health. Not only does it make for greater precision in the quality of information available and the ways in which it is distributed, it also provides important opportunities for engaging stake-holders in decision-making. Effective communication must be informed by an understanding of the factors which influence individual and social responses to risk; the discussion here has attempted to provide an insight into some of these. The continuing challenge is for researchers and those dealing with public health risks, including practitioners, managers, and policy-makers, to build on and take forward the growing amounts of infor-mation we now have on the qualitative dimensions of risk.

## REFERENCES

Adams, J. (1995). *Risk*. UCL Press, London.

Bostrom, A., Fischhoff, B., and Granger Morgan, M. (1992). Characterising mental models of hazardous processes: a methodology and an application to radon. *Journal of Social Issues*, **48**, 85–100.

Combs, B. and Slovic, P. (1979). Newspaper coverage of causes of death. *Journalism Quarterly*, **56**, 837–43.

Commission of the European Communities (1996). *Future noise policy*, (European Commission Green Paper, COM (1996) 540 Final). Office for Official Publications of the European Communities, Luxembourg.

Department of the Environment (1994). *Survey of public attitudes to the environment: England and Wales*. HMSO, London.

Department of Environment/Department of Health (1996). *United Kingdom National Environment Health Action Plan* (Cm3323). HMSO, London.

Department of Health (1997). *Communicating about risks to public health—pointers to good practice*. Department of Health, London. (2nd edition, Stationery Office 1998)

Ferguson, E., Cox, T., Farnsworth, W., Irving, K., and Leiter, M. (1994). Nurses' anxieties about biohazards as a function of context and knowledge. *Journal of Applied Social Psychology*, **24**, 926–40.

Freudenburg, W. R., Coleman, C.-L., Gonzales, J., and Helgeland, C. (1996). Media coverage of hazard events: analyzing the assumptions. *Risk Anaysis*, **16**, 31–42.

Frewer, L. J., Raats, M. M., and Shepherd, R. (1993). Modelling the media: the transmission of risk information in the British quality press. *IMA Journal of Mathematics Applied in Business and Industry*, **5**, 235–47.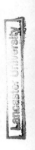

Health Education Authority/Institute for Environment and Health (1997). *Air pollution: what people think about air pollution, their health in general and asthma in particular*. Health Education Authority, London.

Institute for Environment and Health (1997). *IEH report on the non-auditory effects of noise*, Report R10. Institute for Environment and Health, Leicester.

Kasperson, R. E., Renn, O., Slovic, P., Brown, H. S., Emel, J., Goble, R., *et al.* (1988). The social amplification of risk: a conceptual framework. *Risk Analysis*, **8**, 177–87.

Marris, C., Langford, I. and O'Riordan, T. (1996). *Integrating sociological and psychological approaches to public perceptions of environmental risks: detailed results from a questionnaire survey*. Centre for Social and Economic Research on the Global Environment, Norwich.

Renn, O. and Levine, D. (1991). Credibility and trust in risk communication. In *Communicating risks to the public*, (ed. R. E. Kasperson and P. J. M. Stallen), pp. 175–218. Kluwer Academic Publications, The Netherlands.

Royal Society (1992). *Risk: analysis, perception and management*, (2nd edn). The Royal Society, London.

Scott, S. and Freeman, R. (1995). Prevention as a problem of modernity: the example of HIV and AIDS. In *Medicine, health and risk*, (ed. J. Gabe), pp. 151–70. Black-well, Oxford.

Slovic, P. (1987). Perception of risk. *Science*, **236**, 280–5.

Slovic, P. (1993). Perceived risk, trust and democracy. *Risk Analysis*, **13**, 675–82.

UK Government (1998). *Our Healthier Nation—A contract for health* (Cm3852). The Stationery Office, London.

Weigman, O. and Gutterling, J. M. (1995). Risk appraisal and communication—some empirical data from the Netherlands. *Basic Applied Social Psychology*, **16**, 227–49.

# 5 Public health communication and the social amplification of risks: present knowledge and future prospects

Nick Pidgeon, *School of Psychology, University of Wales, Bangor*
Karen Henwood, *Health Policy and Practice, University of East Anglia* and
Bryan Maguire, *Department of Science, Dun Laoghaire Institute of Art Design and Technology*

## Introduction

The question of how and when to engage in systematic communication and dialogue about health risks with the public and other stakeholder groups has today become a central concern of many institutions, including government regulators and administrators. However, the Royal Society study group (Pidgeon *et al.* 1992) has highlighted that while the basic risk perceptions field is a mature one, the social science literature on the matter has remained fragmented, as, for example, between the well-established empirical psychometric and the more theoretically oriented social and cultural approaches to risk. In addition to this, after 20 years of research effort there is currently an extensive debate over the precise implications of the main risk perception research findings for policy (for various commentaries on this, see Okrent and Pidgeon 1998). One view—probably the majority within the social science risk community today—is that the combined findings do offer insights for enriching the knowledge base of scientific decision-making, for aiding in an effective risk communication dialogue, and for further democratizing the risk policy process (National Research Council, 1996; Pidgeon 1998*a*).

The social amplification of risk framework first proposed by Kasperson *et al.* (1988) was conceived initially in an attempt to overcome the theoretical fragmentation of the risk perception and communication field. Their thesis is that certain aspects of hazard events interact with psychological, social, institutional, and cultural processes in ways that might attenuate or intensify perceptions of risk and, through this, shape behaviour. It is claimed that such behavioural responses can in turn generate secondary sociopolitical or economic consequences. There is anecdotal evidence that risk intensification phenomena have occurred in the UK and Europe in recent years, in response both to government and industry attempts to communicate risks to the public, as well as to actual prominent accidents. In the public health domain recent examples include responses to publicity about risks from certain oral contraceptives, and the unfolding BSE crisis which we discuss further below. In other diverse domains, travel patterns altered after both the Lockerbie and King's Cross disasters, and public pressure and a consumer boycott led to the abandonment of Shell's initial plan to dispose of the Brent Spar oil platform in the North Atlantic. Other prominent examples could be readily cited.

Our discussion of the risk amplification model and its implications for public health policy is structured in three sections. In the first, the basic risk amplification framework is outlined. Second, some important caveats which serve to define the boundary conditions for the model are noted. In the third and final section, existing empirical findings are briefly summarized, before exploring some of the future research priorities raised by the discussion.

# The risk amplification framework

In the basic risk amplification model described by Renn (1991), the organizational structure of risk communication within a society comprises sources, transmitters, and receivers, as shown in Fig. 5.1. With much formal risk communication today, primary sources are typically scientific communities and government agencies, while transmitters are dominated by the media, and receivers of information are substructured in the general public. And although the primary flow of information is shown from left to right in Fig. 5.1, feedback can and invariably does occur between the parties in a variety of ways, reflecting the fact noted earlier that risk communication is almost always a process of two-way exchange or dialogue. Figure 5.1 is, of course, a much simplified characterization of a very complex set of relationships: hence, scientists, agency, and media representatives are a part of the public too; the 'general public' itself is not homogeneous but highly differentiated in terms of attitudes towards risk; people actively seek out information, and also receive information and interpretations from other sources significant to them such as family and friends; 'non-experts' can be shown to hold valid local knowledge about aspects of the risk management process (e.g. about the practical circumstances under which a

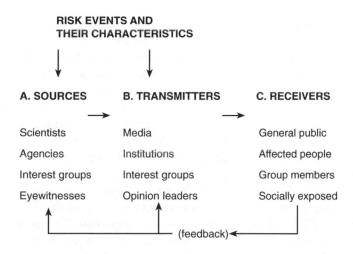

**Fig. 5.1**    Organizational structure of risk communication. (Adapted from Renn (1991).)

particular chemical or food will be used) which will sometimes be over-looked by scientists and other experts; and the sources, transmitters, and receivers are each embedded in their own often very different cultures, which will have a bearing upon how they interpret the meaning of hazards and 'risk'. In addition to this, an often overlooked implication of the model shown in Fig. 5.1 is that, while it is relatively easy to point to the public and media as the originators of problems of risk communication, the sources must also be considered as a key part of the process.

The theoretical foundations of the social amplification framework are developed in Kasperson *et al.* (1988). As well as an integrated framework spanning findings from a wide range of approaches to risk communication and perception, it is also used, more narrowly, to describe the various dynamics of the social processes by which certain hazards and events seen to be relatively low in risk by experts can become a particular focus of concern and sociopolitical activity within a society (risk intensification), while other more serious hazards receive comparatively less attention (risk attenuation). Examples of public health hazards subject to social attenuation of risk perceptions might include naturally occurring radon gas or smoking. The model assumes that 'risk events', which might be actual or hypothesized characteristics of hazards (including accidents and incidents), will be largely irrelevant or localized in their impact unless they are communicated to someone (Renn 1991). The social amplification framework holds that, as a key part of that communication process, risk events and their characteristics become portrayed through various risk signals (images, signs, and symbols) which in turn interact with a wide range of psychological, social, institutional, or cultural processes in ways that intensify or attenuate perceptions of risk. Within such a framework, risk experience is defined through the interaction between the objective harms attached to a risk event and the social and cultural processes which shape interpretations of that event.

The authors adopt the metaphor of amplification from classical communication theory, using this to describe the way in which risk signals are received, interpreted, and passed on by a variety of social agents. In the first stage of their model, signals are held to undergo predictable transformations as they are filtered through various social and individual 'amplification stations'. Such transformations can involve an increase or decrease in the volume of information about an event, selection to heighten the salience of certain aspects of a message important for that particular amplification station, or reinterpretation and elaboration of the available symbols and images, leading to other interpretations and responses by subsequent recipients of secondary messages. Amplification stations can include both individuals and institutions; for example, scientists or scientific institutions, reporters, and the mass media, politicians and government agencies, or other stakeholder groups and their members. For social stations of amplification, intensification or attenuation of aspects of risk signals ought to be predictable from such things as institutional culture and structure. For individual risk amplifiers this derives from such things as prior attitudes, demographic characteristics, group memberships, and world-view.

In a second stage of the framework, directed primarily at risk intensification processes, it is argued that social amplification can also account for the observation that some events will lead to spreading 'ripples' of secondary consequences, which may go far beyond the initial impact of the event, and may even impinge upon initially unrelated hazards. Such secondary consequences include market impacts (perhaps through consumer avoidance of a product or related products), calls for regulatory constraints, litigation, community opposition, loss of credibility and trust, stigmatization of a facility or community, and investor flight

As a brief example, consider the BSE crisis, and in particular the impact in March 1996 of public confirmation of a new variant of CJD with the implication that a link might exist—now supported by subsequent evidence —between the disease in cattle and humans (see Chapter 7). As noted above, social intensification of risk perceptions appears to have been one feature of the recent history of this crisis (although one could also argue, perhaps more controversially and with the benefits of hindsight, that prior to the March 1996 announcement there had not been *enough* public concern over this issue, a point to which the discussion returns later). There is at the moment only fragmented empirical evidence concerning the precise impacts of this event on perceptions in the UK and continental Europe—and undoubtedly a need now to conduct systematic research on this key question to support future public health risk communication as the uncertainties still surrounding this disease unfold over the coming years. What is clear, however, is that the primary (stage I) impacts from this attempt at risk communication in March 1996 have involved an intense level of media scrutiny coupled with a rapid and radical reframing of public understanding of the risk and its characteristics. The stage II impacts have been many and varied, including: a complex set of changes in food consumption patterns (in the UK, other European states, and worldwide); further mistrust of official sources of information about food production and generalization of this to other food technology issues, e.g. the safety of genetically modified organisms (Grove-White *et al.* 1997; Chapters 11 and 12) to the extent that a very significant effort—going well beyond mere 'public relations'—will be required to restore public confidence in the handling of food safety matters; and disagreement at intergovernmental level regarding the appropriate risk management measures to adopt. As Tennant (1997) observes, the March 1996 announcement, preceded as it was by a history of messages that beef was 'safe', probably triggered a number of outrage factors identified from psychometric research as important to heightened risk perceptions: i.e. feelings of *involuntariness* because consumers do not always know which foods contain beef products, *lack of control* over the risk, worries about a *dreaded* disease, and significant residual *uncertainty* over the future impacts upon society. To this can be added several institutional issues, including the question of *blame* for what is clearly a classic organizational/technological failure of foresight (Turner and Pidgeon (1997) provide a general model to characterize the build-up to such failures), and the *undermining of trust* because of an apparent reversal in the government position regarding beef safety. As we note below, it was probably not any one of these factors alone, but several in combination, which galvanized the large social responses to this event. It is clear also that the scientific uncertainties of the case were at that time more fluid and ill-structured than could be captured in any simple safe/unsafe characterization —raising a serious dilemma for current risk communication about this issue.

## Critiques of the model

Despite its *prima facie* plausibility, the risk amplification metaphor has not been without its critics. Therefore, we note in this section a set of important caveats that help us to explore the boundary conditions of the model. One drawback is that the framework may be too general to subject to any direct empirical test, particularly one of outright falsification. Its originators now concede (Renn 1991; Kasperson 1992) that social amplification may not represent a theory in the classical sense, but rather serves as a useful analytic tool for describing and organizing relevant phenomena, for exploring and integrating relationships between rival constituent theories concerning risk perception and its communication, and for deriving new hypotheses about the societal processing of risk signals (the latter could then, in principle at least, be tested directly). It can also be argued, despite the recognition of important mechanisms and routes of feedback as depicted in Fig. 5.1 above, that the communications-engineering model on which the approach is founded places the dominant emphasis upon too simple a conceptualization of risk communication, as a *one-way* transfer of information; i.e. from risk events and sources, through transmitters, and then onto receivers. Pidgeon *et al.* (1992) argue that the development of social risk perceptions is always likely to be the product of more interactive processes between the parties to any risk communication.

A further point concerns the two-stage nature of the original model, and the existing evidence to support each stage. Stage I posits that signals from risk events become transformed to influence perceptions of risk and, through this, first-order behavioural responses. There is now a relatively extensive set of findings from the risk perception literature to suggest this is the case, although much remains to be done to investigate the specific contexts under which intensification or attenuation will occur. Stage II involves a direct link between amplification of risk perceptions and secondary consequences such as calls for stricter regulation, stigmatization of technologies, market impacts, and a generalization of response to other similar risk events and hazards. In many respects it is this stage II which is the most important for policy, given the potential here for large health and economic impacts, but concrete stage II effects remain very much an hypothesis based upon fragmented evidence, rather than one which is supported by systematic empirical research.

While much has been made of the negative consequences of risk *intensification* (which for obvious reasons tend to be the most visible), it is also clearly the case that *attenuation* of risk signals can be equally undesirable, depending upon one's standpoint regarding issues of risk management and the nature of the hazard. Kasperson and Kasperson (1990) have developed a theoretical analysis of the reasons why serious hazards might systematically become 'hidden' (e.g. where they affect marginal groups, conflict with deeply held values other than safety, or where there are institutional constraints upon the extent of formal risk assessment). And we also know from research over the past 20 years on the organizational origins of serious safety failures in complex social-technical systems (of which modern public health care—capable of generating a wide range of unintended iatrogenic hazards—is one example) that they tend to have long 'incubation periods', where a number of initially seemingly unrelated contributory errors and decisions combine in unanticipated ways over time to circumvent or disable the available safety systems, generating a situation where a disaster is 'waiting to happen' (Turner and Pidgeon 1997). What is more, the organization of modern systems of production and distribution means that the consequences of an error (say bacterial contamination of food, or poorly sterilized hospital supplies) that occurs at an early stage in the production system may lead to impacts that initially lie hidden while they are being distributed widely across an exposed population.

Organizational 'failure of foresight' is almost always implicated in such safety breakdowns too, as the early warning messages and signs of danger that are available are missed, or interpreted as giving little or no cause for concern. This might be because the problem falls beyond an organization's area of immediate or legal remit, because of failure to assemble fragmented information, reluctance to take seriously the views of dissenters and 'whistle-bowers' in possession of useful information at variance with the received view, because of culturally limited vision within large bureaucracies or isolated policy-making groups, or through institutionally generated ignorance and secrecy (Manning 1998; Pidgeon 1998b). Countering such bounded vision is no easy matter, and requires both the ability to exercise critical scrutiny of the existing assumptions upon which current understanding of the world and its hazards are founded (something which might be termed 'safety imagination'), together with the political will to counteract the power dynamics of organizations and small groups which tend to marginalize dissent and place other blocks on effective organizational learning (Pidgeon 1997).

It follows from the above that some risk amplification effects might be entirely desirable, as when sufficient public and political pressure for action to tackle a previously neglected (attenuated) but very serious hazard is finally generated. To take an example from health and safety legislation, Behrens (1983) gives an account of the legislative changes that followed the fire which began in the eighth floor workrooms of one of New York's 'loft' clothing factories at the Triangle Shirtwaist Company in 1911. By the year of the disaster, over half of the city's 500 000 workers worked above the seventh floor—many in poorly maintained and equipped buildings, and all beyond the reach of effective fire department rescue. The fire led to the deaths of 146 clothing workers, many of whom became trapped and attempted to escape by jumping from the upper stories of the burning building. Although, according to Behrens, the initial public outrage at the factory management's disregard for safety eventually subsided, in the short term it was the stimulus for much needed reform of fire and workplace safety regulations in the city. Behrens concludes that 'in the immediate aftermath of major disasters, groups and individuals interested in reform are given unexpected opportunities to effect reforms that normally would take years'.

Finally, a number of criticisms have also been raised of the amplification metaphor itself. The term 'amplification' is typically associated, in more common usage, with the intensification of signals, and hence it can be argued that the framework incorporates an implicit semantic bias. It is clear, however, from our discussion above that the detailed proposal can describe both the social processes that attenuate signals about hazards, as well as those involved in intensification. A second, more serious criticism of the metaphor, is that it might be taken to imply that there exists a baseline or 'true' risk that can be readily attached to risk events, which is then *distorted* in some way by the social processes of amplification. It is quite clear that the proponents of the framework do not wish to imply that such a single true baseline always and unproblematically exists. Their conceptualization of the amplification process in terms of transformation of signs, symbols, and images is compatible with the view that, while hazards certainly do have real consequences (either direct impacts or secondary ones through stage-II effects), all knowledge about risk entails some element of social construction and interpretation; and the fact that experts and public sometimes disagree about risks is compatible with the claim of the model that different groups and cultures filter and make salient different aspects of an event. Without wanting to open up the contentious debate on 'objective' versus 'subjective' risk, which so troubled the Royal Society five years ago,[1] anybody who has attempted serious risk analysis will know that even with relatively well-defined hazards there is a range of different risk indicators one might use for communicating relevant information to others, and that in many of the highly ill-structured and heavily politicized settings where amplification and attenuation are most likely to occur the uncertainties are too wide to state definitively what 'the risk' is anyway (Pidgeon *et al.* 1992). Perhaps the more important point, for practical risk communication purposes, is to seek an understanding of the dynamics of change in risk perceptions and behaviour: why and how rapid changes in public understanding and framing of risk, as

---

1. Horlick-Jones (1998) provides an illuminating commentary on this debate (see also Adams 1995). As the current first author was one of the chief protagonists, I should make clear that my own conclusion on this issue was that *all* understandings of risk—both expert and lay—inevitably involve some degree of judgement and interpretation. *However,* this does not necessarily imply a disabling position of philosophical relativism (any view on risk is as good as any other), but rather raises the key questions of how we bring the best *quality* judgement, the most *relevant* information, and the most *effective* analytic/decision process to bear upon the particular problem at hand?

has occurred with BSE, might occur in certain contexts and at critical moments in history (or alternatively, for 'hidden hazards', not occur).

# The empirical base

In this penultimate section we very briefly note existing empirical findings and their broad conclusions. Since the framework is by design inclusive, the literature concerning general phenomena of relevance to the social amplification of risk is potentially a very large one indeed. There is now a wide range of evidence to draw upon regarding the interaction of risk events and signals with social, institutional, and cultural processes. These include work on demographic and occupational affiliation, attitudes and belief salience, world-views of risk, and cultural influences (for overviews see Pidgeon and Beattie 1998; Pidgeon *et al.* 1992). Regarding specific studies of social amplification, Slovic *et al.* (1984) first proposed that certain hazardous events might hold a 'signal value'. They report that hazards such as nuclear power—which are capable of evoking strong feelings of 'dread' and are seen as relatively 'unknown' are judged to have high signal value in terms of serving as a warning sign for society, providing new information about the probability that similar or even more destructive mishaps might occur with this type of activity. Such high signal value might also be linked to the potential for second-order amplification effects.

Kasperson and colleagues have conducted two direct empirical studies, one quantitative and one qualitative, of social amplification and its effects (Kasperson 1992). The quantitative study involved a statistical analysis of 128 US hazard events, including biocidal hazards, persistent/delayed hazards, rare catastrophes, common causes of death, global diffuse hazards, and natural hazards. Data were collected on the actual volume of media coverage each received, and then related to judgements made by experts and student panels of the physical consequences, risk perceptions, public response, and the potential for second-order societal impacts of each event. A number of findings emerged, particularly that social amplification processes are as important as direct physical consequences in determining potential socio-economic effects. Hence, a risk assessment that is based solely upon direct *physical* consequences might underestimate the full range of consequences of an event. Among Kasperson's conclusions from this study are the following:

1.  There is a high degree of 'rationality' in how society responds to hazards, e.g. volume of press coverage is roughly proportional to first-order physical consequences, and risk perceptions incorporate aspects of human exposure and management performance.

2. Extent of exposure to the direct consequences of a hazard has more effect on risk perceptions and potential social group mobilization than do injuries and fatalities.

3. The contention that public perception mirrors media coverage needs further careful empirical study; no psychometric variable—except the ubiquitous 'dread'—correlated with the extent of media coverage once the extent of damage was controlled.

4. The roles of risk signals and blame attributable to poor or negligent risk management seemed particularly important concerns.

The qualitative study by Kasperson (1992) yielded complementary findings. Here, six events—all but one involving some form of nuclear hazard—were studied as in-depth cases. Issues explored included physical impacts, information flow, social group mobilization, and secondary (stage-II) consequences. Conclusions from the qualitative case studies included:

1. Heavy media coverage may not by itself herald risk amplification or secondary effects. Again it appears that trust may be a critical issue mediating this, as is perceived management handling of events.

2. The cases pointed to layering of attenuation/intensification effects across different groups and in time, pointing to more complex and dynamic processes than implied by the basic 'amplification' model.

3. Following on from the first point, it is suggested that several factors need to be present in combination (e.g. media coverage plus the focused attention from a local interest group, or an accident plus prior suspicions of mismanagement) to generate what Kasperson terms 'take off' of an issue.

4. The economic benefits associated with risks appear to be a source of attenuation.

## Concluding comments and new directions

Given the overarching nature of the risk amplification model, we briefly conclude by using the discussion so far as a pointer to a number of critical, unexplored issues for risk communication within the UK and European context.

1. A first point is that much of the existing empirical work on risk communication and the social amplification of risk reflects North American experience. There is clearly a need to conduct basic investigation of the transferability of the model and findings with respect to

current health issues in Europe—for example, whether the theoretical concepts of trust, blame, and responsibility for risk management play as strong a role here (or in the same ways) as is accorded in the US—as well as the aspects of the European cultural context which uniquely shape health risk communication and associated amplification effects. As noted earlier, Fig. 5.1 cautions us against taking the simplistic view that attributes risk communication problems solely to the audience alone. Understanding the standpoints and amplification rules of all three sets of actors, along with some actors which we might not have anticipated (e.g. internet newsgroups), will all be critical to this process.

2.  The dominant methodological approach to risk perceptions arose from, and in the main has continued to follow, the traditional quantitative paradigm of psychology, and this strategy has yielded a range of valuable findings. However, research that is fully culturally sensitive needs also to explore, in some considerable depth, the meanings and interpretations which respondents themselves place upon images, signs, and signals relating to events in their wider cultural and historical context (Henwood and Pidgeon 1992). This is likely to involve an emphasis in the future upon work of a more qualitative nature alongside the traditional quantitative approaches to risk perception research.

3.  It is clear from the discussion so far that we should not simply seek to pathologize the most obvious instances of extreme intensification and attenuation in understandings of risk. The reality of risk communication is far less straightforward than this. The impacts of attenuation and intensification effects can bring both positive and negative consequences, and this in turn will depend upon the perspective from which a hazard and its history is viewed. Again, Fig. 5.1 is useful in alerting us to the potentially different standpoints which might be taken on any issue, and we now need some philosophical reflection on why events might be framed as negative, and from whose perspective, and when alternatively they might be seen as 'desired'.

4.  We have noted the fact that social amplification of risk should not be viewed as a theory, yielding simple and direct predictions, but as an analytic framework. Taken together with the inherent complexity of risk communication issues, it is clear that the framework cannot be expected to yield simple or direct predictions regarding which issues are likely to be the subject of intensification/attenuation effects in advance. A similar problem—which has in part epistemological, and in part practical roots —is met when researchers attempt to use knowledge of the human and organizational causes from past technological incidents and disasters to predict the likelihood of future failures of foresight (Pidgeon 1997).

*Ex post* it is always easy to demonstrate that 'X management decision' or 'Y human error' led inexorably towards failure, or that 'Z was a signal of impending disaster' that should have been heeded at the time. Such statements are almost always hindsight judgements, which overlook the considerable uncertainty and noise which inevitably surround proactive risk management decisions, and make past events seem far more certain than they were to those involved at the time. In seeking to overcome this very real constraint on prediction, accident researchers have sought to evaluate ongoing risk management against a range of broad holistic indicators of failure potential (Wagenaar *et al.* 1994). In a similar way, and as Kasperson (1996) comments, knowledge of the factors likely to lead to amplification effects, and the contexts in which they might operate, could possibly be used as a *screening device* for evaluating the potential impacts of health risk communications in a particular domain.

5. Following on from the previous point, and the empirical findings of Kasperson (1992), it appears that both dynamic changes in framing or 'take-off' of risk issues, as well as the continued existence of attenuated or hidden hazards, will often involve the interaction of several critical factors. We do not as yet know if there is any systematic pattern to the factors which are most likely to interact in any given context. Pursuing the analogy with incubating disasters a little further, it would be no surprise to find that in both cases some of the contributory factors will have been in place for a considerable period of time. BSE again appears to be a paradigm example of this in the public health domain. The final lesson then is that the design of any risk communication needs to take as much account of what came before it, as it does of the message content or objectives to be achieved in the present.

## REFERENCES

Adams, J. (1995). *Risk*. University College London Press, London.

Behrens, E. G. (1983). The Triangle Shirtwaist Company fire of 1911: a lesson in legislative manipulation. *Texas Law Review*, **62**, 361–87.

Grove-White, R., Mcnaghten, P., Mayer, S., and Wynne, B. (1997). *Uncertain world: genetically modified organisms, food and public attitudes in Britain*. Centre for the Study of Environmental Change, Lancaster University, Lancaster.

Henwood, K. L. and Pidgeon, N. F. (1992). Qualitative research and psychological theorizing. *The British Journal of Psychology*, **83**, 97–111.

Horlick-Jones, T. (1998). Meaning and contextualisation in risk assessment. *Reliability Engineering and System Safety*, **59**, 79–89.

Kasperson, R. E. (1992). The social amplification of risk: progress in developing an integrative framework. In *Social theories of risk* (ed. S. Krimsky and D. Golding), pp. 153–178. Praeger, Westport CT.

Kasperson, R. E. (1996). *Risk communication and the social amplification of risk*. ILGRA/HSE seminar, 19 November, London.

Kasperson, R. E. and Kasperson, J. X. (1990). Hidden hazards. In *Acceptable evidence: science and values in hazard management* (ed. D. Mayo and R. Hollander), pp. 9–28. Oxford University Press, Oxford.

Kasperson, R. E., Renn, O., Slovic, P., Brown, H. S., Emel, J., Goble, R., *et al.* (1988). The social amplification of risk: a conceptual framework. *Risk Analysis*, **8**, 177–87.

Manning, P. (1998). Information, socio-technical disasters and politics. *Journal of Contingencies and Crisis Management*, **6**, 84–7.

National Research Council (1996). *Understanding risk: informing decisions in a democratic society*. National Academy Press, Washington DC.

Okrent, D. and Pidgeon, N. F. (1998). Risk assessment versus risk perception. Special single issue of *Reliability Engineering and System Safety*, **59**, 1–159.

Pidgeon, N. F. (1997). The limits to safety? Culture, politics, learning and man-made disasters. *Journal of Contingencies and Crisis Management*, **5**, 1–14.

Pidgeon, N. F. (1998a) Risk assessment, risk values and the social science programme: why we do need risk perception research. *Reliability Engineering and System Safety*, **59**, 5–15.

Pidgeon, N. F. (1998b) Shaking the kaleidoscope of disasters research—a reply. *Journal of Contingencies and Crisis Management*, **6**, 97–101.

Pidgeon, N. F. and Beattie, J. (1998). The psychology of risk and uncertainty. In *Handbook of environmental risk assessment and management,* (ed. P. Calow), pp. 289–318. Blackwell Science, Oxford.

Pidgeon, N. F., Hood, C., Jones, D., Turner, B. A., and Gibson, R. (1992). Risk perception. In *Risk: analysis, perception and management*, pp. 89–134. The Royal Society, London.

Renn, O. (1991). Risk communication and the social amplification of risk. In *Communicating risks to the public* (ed. R. E. Kasperson and P. J. M. Stallen), pp. 287–323. Kluwer, Dordrecht.

Slovic, P., Lichtenstein, S., and Fischhoff, B. (1984). Modeling the societal impact of fatal accidents. *Management Science*, **30**, 464–74.

Tennant, D. R. (1997). The communication of risks and the risks of communication. *Risk, Decision and Policy*, **2**, 147–53.

Turner, B. A. and Pidgeon, N. F. (1997). *Man-made disasters*, (2nd edn). Butterworth-Heinemann, Oxford.

Wagenaar, W. A., Groeneweg, J., Hudson, P. T. W., and Reason, J. T. (1994). Promoting safety in the oil industry. *Ergonomics*, **37**, 1999–2013.

# PART 2

---

# Lessons from prominent cases

## Preface to Part 2

Prominent risk communication episodes have already made their appearance in Part 1 of the book, though mainly to illustrate particular points in passing. The following chapters look at specific cases in more depth, and seek lessons for those seeking to communicate with the public about health risks.

We start with some episodes that achieved national prominence in the UK—and in some cases worldwide. The responses to Necrotizing Fasciitis (the infamous 'flesh-eating bug') and *E. coli* food infection are discussed by Professor Hugh Pennington, whose report on the latter can be seen as a landmark in British food safety policy. Robert Maxwell provides an account of BSE/CJD as a food safety issue, concentrating not so much on the risk communication 'outputs'—discussed by many other contributors—as on the scientific perceptions and risk assessment on which policy was based. The last two contributions each draw general conclusions from a wide range of episodes. Ronan Lyons and Dorothy Wright bring to bear their experiences within a public health team based in Wales, dealing with issues ranging from shipwreck to sewage. Finally, Tony Taig's chapter draws on an extended comparative study of risk communication practice across government, encompassing a series of case studies taking in road safety, infant feeding, land use planning, and agricultural practice.

# 6 The media and trust: *E. coli* and other cases

Hugh Pennington
*Department of Medical Microbiology, University of Aberdeen*

## Introduction

It is a truth universally acknowledged that the media play a central—often defining—role in risk communication. Thus it has been pointed out by Reilly and Miller (1997) that not only are there major debates about the media and its damaging impact on the 'gullible' public, but it is accepted that it also has effects on industry, government, pressure groups, and a host of other categories of organization. These workers have gone so far as to claim that it was likely that the Food Safety Act was born partly out of media coverage of *Salmonella* and *Listeria*. This claim echoes the view of Nelkin (1989) that the

> 'media coverage of risk events reverberates through the political system, forcing responses from politicians. By calling public attention to an issue, the media may affect the nature of regulation, the course of litigation or the direction of research and development'.

In this paper I report the pilot results of an analysis of personal interactions with the media during two events: the 1994 flesh-eating bug/necrotizing fasciitis episode, and the events that occurred during and after the 1996 outbreak of *E. coli* O157 food poisoning in central Scotland. The justification for presenting what might appear to be nothing more than a self-seeking autobiographical account is that at least by my own estimation I had significant interactions with the media in both events. In addition it can be hubristically claimed that a study of this type follows the historic tradition of opportunistic self-analysis exemplified by John Dalton and his colour blindness. Most importantly, by reporting on the direct relationships between the media and one of its sources, it is hoped that this account will provide information that can be used to get a better understanding of the factors that determine topic selection (one of the three aspects of news production which combine to affect the final media product, the others being the treatment and the telling of the story (Hartley 1982)). I hope it will also provide information that can be used to test hypotheses and notions about these factors, such as those identified by Galtung and Ruge (1973)—negative characteristics, rarity, interpretability within the dominant cultural framework, personal relevance to reader, listener, or viewer, and referability to things affecting specific, particularly named, individuals—and the notion that in order to maximize reader numbers newspapers concentrate on 'human interest' stories, which show a world composed of individuals whose lives are 'governed by luck, fate, and chance', and which portray life as a lottery (Curran *et al.* 1980).

A quantitative approach is adopted where possible and a review of the time-course of events is presented rather than a purely anecdotal account with superimposed opinion. First- and second-hand accounts of this latter type are being published more frequently (Haslam and Boyman 1994; Kitzinger and Reilly 1997). They often focus on the published outcomes (or lack of them) of interactions between sources and media reporters. Detailed analyses of the media coverage of the necrotizing fasciitis episode and the 1996 *E. coli* O157 outbreak have not been done and so media outputs will receive only limited consideration in this Chapter. This will be illustrative rather than comprehensive.

The circumstances which led to my involvement in the events described here were as follows. In 1992 I obtained funding to conduct research on *Streptococcus pyogenes*, the cause of scarlet fever, primarily to develop new molecular techniques for strain typing to better follow their spread, and in particular to test the idea current in the USA at that time that infections caused by certain virulent strains of this organism were occurring more frequently. My name was on a list held by the British Medical Association of experts willing to talk to the media, with streptococci being listed as one of my interests. In 1992 I had also set up the Scottish Reference Laboratory for *E. coli* O157 after Aberdeen had been awarded a contract for this by the Scottish Health Service Central Services Agency on the initiative of the Scottish Health Service. Before 1994 my contacts with the media had been restricted to a scripted interview on Children's Hour in 1955, intermittent contacts with the local morning and evening daily papers, and most importantly, fairly regular participation in an intellectual chat show on BBC Radio Scotland—nearly always from a self-operated studio in Aberdeen, with the host in Glasgow and other participants in studios elsewhere. This had given me experience in radio techniques and a degree of self-confidence with this medium—not because the producers said how much they enjoyed my contribution (they do this to everybody) but because I was asked back.

During both the 1994 necrotizing fasciitis and the 1996 *E. coli* O157 episodes I interacted with the media in the same way—essentially by reacting positively to all bids for telephone interviews, interviews in my office/ laboratory, and interviews at the three local broadcasting stations (BBC, Grampian TV, and independent radio, all located within 5 minutes driving time of my laboratory and 5 minutes walking distance from my home). All telephone calls were logged. I made no approaches to the media myself. In being cooperative with the media it might be thought that this behaviour was unusual for a scientist. I take comfort by quoting Lewenstein (1995) who has pointed out that the notion that scientists do not like to cooperate with the media is a myth, concluding that 'virtually every systematic attempt to look at this question has shown that scientists are extremely willing to work with the press' and that 'though it may serve the traditional norms of science to declare that science should be communicated only among scientific peers, both scientific institutions and individual scientists have long recognized the value of communicating with the public'.

Public relations professionals from three institutions were also involved from time to time. Three press conferences about *E. coli* O157 in 1997 and the many interviews that occurred immediately after the two ministerial ones were arranged by the Scottish Office; they are not considered in this paper and are not included in the quantitative analyses. Contacts with the university press office were infrequent and restricted to them passing on media bids. The NHS Trust, in which my office and the Reference Laboratory are located, followed to a degree the familiar path of trying to 'exercise communication controls' (Haslam and Boyman 1994), in this case by insisting on prior knowledge of the appearance of TV cameras in the department.

# Necrotizing fasciitis

The clinical events which precipitated this episode have been described by Cartwright *et al.* (1995). Two patients from the Stroud area of Gloucestershire underwent elective surgery in the same operating theatre, one on 4 February and the other on 7 February 1994. Both developed necrotizing fasciitis. Subsequent cases of necrotizing fasciitis in west Gloucestershire presented on 18 February, 7 April, 15 April, and 11 May. One of these patients resided in Stroud and the others lived 1, 15, and 40 km away. Two died. The cluster of cases first received media attention outside the local area at the beginning of May, when the BBC South of England health correspondent broadcast a radio item about them. The story was run by the Press Association on 11 May and attracted the attention of a *Daily Sport* journalist. This paper carried out a report about it on the 13 May, replacing its usual front page sex story with the headline *BUG THAT EATS YOU ALIVE* and, in lower case, *Killer virus scoffs three*. Two weeks later the story had spread worldwide, with items being carried on Canadian television and Australian radio. Its end was marked by the appearance of leaders in the *Lancet*, the *British Medial Journal, Nature*, and *Science* in early June. The acute microbiology and epidemiology investigations were handled by the Public Health Laboratory Service. Its London HQ handled about 1000 enquiries during the incident and its Gloucester laboratory received 200 requests for information.

The number of media outlets (newspapers, radio programmes, television stations) telephoning me for microbiological information between 12 and 28 May 1994 is shown in Fig. 6.1. Enquiries from newspapers occurred in three phases. The first enquiry (*The Daily Sport*) was followed by another and then by about a week of silence. The number of calls then rose rapidly, peaking on Monday 23 May. A slow fall during the remainder of the week was marked by the replacement of calls from daily publications by those from Sunday papers.

Television and radio enquiries lagged behind those from the press, peaking on Wednesday 25 May. A graph showing the cumulative number of calls is shown in Fig. 6.2. It shows an S-shaped, or logistic curve.

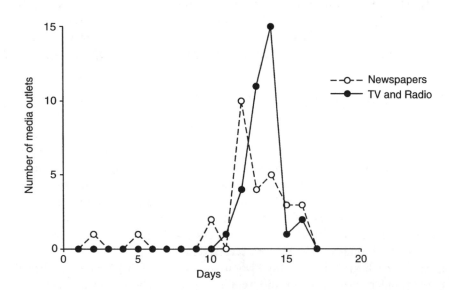

**Fig. 6.1**   Number of media outlets telephoning between 12 May (day 1) and 27 May 1994. (○) Newspapers; (●) radio prgrammes and television channels (with permission).

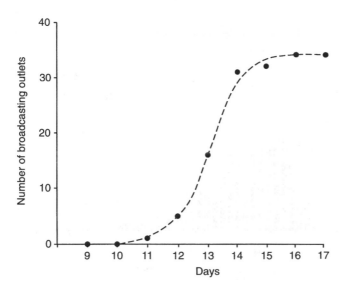

**Fig. 6.2** Cumulative number of broadcasting outlets (radio programmes, television channels) telephoning between 20 May (day 9) and 27 May 1994 (with permission).

# The Central Scotland *E. coli* O157 outbreak

On the afternoon of Friday 22 November 1996 the Public Health Department of Lanarkshire Health Board became aware of several cases of infection with *E. coli* O157 in residents of Wishaw in the central belt of Scotland. By the evening, histories from confirmed or suspected cases indicated that 14 of the 15 patients had consumed food obtained directly or indirectly from J. Barr and Son, Butchers of Wishaw. Although outwardly a small, local butcher with adjacent bakery shop, the business was involved at the time of the outbreak in a substantial wholesale and retail trade involving the production and distribution of raw and cooked meats and bakery products from the Wishaw premises. The epidemic curve for the outbreak (Fig. 6.3) shows that the number of suspected or confirmed infections increased dramatically from its onset.

Epidemiological and subsequent microbiological evidence shows that the outbreak comprised several separate but related incidents relating to a lunch (attended by more than 70 frail elderly people) held in Wishaw Parish Church Hall on 17 November, a birthday party held in the Cascade Public House on 23 November, and retail sales in Lanarkshire and Forth Valley. The outbreak was declared over on Monday 20 January 1997, although further deaths occurred following prolonged illness. The final tally of cases

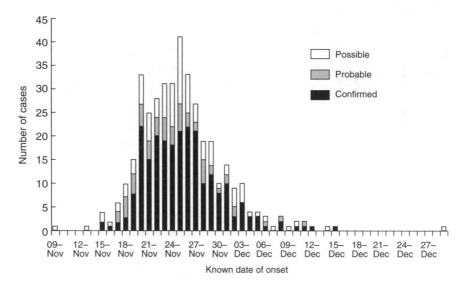

**Fig. 6.3**   *E. coli* O157 central Scotland outbreak epidemic curve by date of onset of diarrhoea (Pennington 1997, with permission).

was 501 (the largest ever outbreak of infection with the organism in the UK). There were admitted to hospital 127 people, of whom 13 required dialysis. There were 20 deaths (all adults) associated with the outbreak—the highest number associated with an outbreak of *E. coli* O157 infection in the world.

On November 28 1996 the Secretary of State for Scotland announced the establishment of an Expert Group under my chairmanship with a remit 'to examine the circumstances which led to the outbreak in the central belt of Scotland and to advise [him] on the implications for food safety and the general lessons to be learned'. In early 1997 a further outbreak of infection with *E. coli* O157 occurred in a nursing home in Tayside and the group was asked to take account of this in its deliberations and of other outbreaks which also occurred in the Borders and Lothian. The Group convened from the beginning of December 1996 until the end of March 1997. An interim report with recommendations was submitted to the Secretary of State on 31 December 1996 and on 15 January 1997 he responded to it in the House of Commons. The final report was submitted at the end of March and published, with the Government's response, on 8 April 1997.

Before the Wishaw outbreak, media enquiries to me about *E. coli* O157 during 1996 occurred at a level ranging from one to six per month. Eighteen of the 31 enquiries were from Scottish organizations. At the beginning of November the TV programme 'Newsnight' came to my department to film the work of a visiting Public Health Laboratory Service staff member as part of an item about the fiftieth anniversary of the Service, and BBC Scotland TV was planning with us a programme about the transmission of *E. coli* O157 to shepherds at lambing. Filming took place in the department on 28 November, the day when the establishment of the Expert Group was announced.

The number of telephone enquiries from the media about *E. coli* O157 during and following the outbreak is shown in Fig. 6.4. Calls are plotted day by day, starting on 25 November 1996 (day 1) and finishing on16 July 1997 (day 230). On nine occasions enquiries peaked at 10 or more per day. The first peak, labelled (a), reflected media activity on the day of the announcement of the Expert Group. One peak (b) coincided with the meeting at the Scottish Office at which the composition of the group was decided and five peaks (c, d, e, f, and h) occurred on the day before the meetings of the Expert Group. Media pressure was particularly sustained just before and on the day of the meeting at which the report was finalized (peak h). The largest peak of all—36 enquiries on 6 March 1997 (g)—was linked to the leaking to the press of the first draft of the Swann report, a review by the Meat Hygiene Service of abattoir hygiene practice conducted in 1995. Highly critical of aspects of abattoir practice, the report underwent significant drafting changes and was eventually put into the public domain in a low-key way in June 1996. Much of the substantial press coverage of 6 March, and that which followed, focused on the actions of the Meat Hygiene Service, government departments, and ministers. My input started with a call from the radio 'Today' programme at about 7.20 am asking whether I knew about the report in any of its versions. My comment that 'I hadn't been shown any of them, and that I was not pleased', became part of the story. The final peak of interest on 2 June (peak i) coincided with the deaths of two elderly women from *E. coli* O157 infection, one a victim of the central Scotland outbreak. Of the total of 557 enquiries, 159 were from television, 126 from radio, 130 from the four Scottish broadsheets (*Press and Journal* (Aberdeen), *Courier* (Dundee), *Herald* (Glasgow), and *Scotsman* (Edinburgh)), 66 from London broadsheets, 29 from tabloids, 20 from science journals, 12 from trade journals, 13 from press agencies, and one each from the *Lancaster Guardian* and the *West Highland Free Press*.

# Discussion

The 'fright factors' and 'media triggers' listed in the Department of Health (1997) document *Pointers to good practice*, are a useful starting point in analyses of the two episodes described here. As a discrete short-lived event, the necrotizing fasciitis episode clearly differs markedly from the events

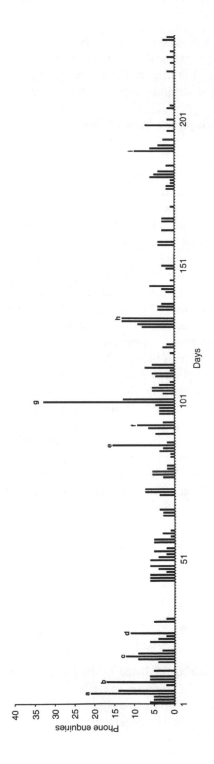

**Fig. 6.4** Number of telephone calls from media organizations between 25 November 1996 (day 1) and 16 July 1997 (day 230).

surrounding the *E. coli* O157 outbreak. Thus, long before that event the media were already paying a good deal of attention to food safety issues and, in Scotland in particular, to *E. coli* O157 as news stories in their own right, whereas the necrotizing fasciitis story appeared and disappeared with a dynamic not unlike an epidemic caused by a virus or a bacterium. It even had a long incubation period. Rather than an outbreak of infection, it was an outbreak of media interest. It scored highly in fright factors, particularly clinical ones. Thus, its acquision seemed *involuntary* because it attacked victims at random, and its distribution was *inequitable*—why so many victims at Stroud, which also had had the misfortune between 1981 and 1986 to be the centre of a meningitis epidemic with more than 60 cases and two deaths? It was *inescapable* because risk factors appeared to be poorly defined, and it was *novel* because its clustering seemed to defy explanation. It caused *irreversible* damage through massive tissue loss, and caused death in a *dreadful* way—'*Bug that eats you alive*' (*The Daily Sport*). Its victims were *identifiable*. It also scored highly in the *human interest* and *visual impact* media triggers, with *powerful images* being conveyed by text, e.g. '*Thank God I'M FAT*' (*Take a Break*), '*BUG EATS HUMAN FLESH*' (*Sunday Mail*).

It is probable that the coming together of all these features accounted for its selection by the media, its strength as a story, and, in part, its persistence. This was also aided by the discovery and description of previously unreported cases by journalists (the media were able to find a number of victims or relatives of victims willing to speak about their experiences—photographs of at least seven have been published and television programmes about two have been made, a creditable tally considering the rarity of the disease), by the raising of uncertainties about its incidence, and by the rehearsal of arguments for and against notification.

The dynamics of media interest in necrotizing fasciitis and the shift of interest from newspapers to broadcasting can be analysed both in terms of the bureaucratic setting which produced it and its mathematical epidemiology. Thus, journalists make extensive use of media organizations other than their own in determining what is news. In a study of crime reporting, Fishman (1981) showed that this mutual dependence between different branches of the media is an important factor in encouraging the spread of a news theme through the community of a news organization, in his case often converting a crime *theme* into a crime *wave*. There is a clear similarity between such events and the spread of necrotizing fasciitis as a news theme and its conversion thereby into an 'outbreak'. In terms of its mathematics, it is highly probable that the basic principles governing the spread of a news theme and the spread of an infectious agent during an epidemic are the same. The course of the latter is governed by the mass-action principle. This indicates that the rate of spread is proportional to the product of the density of susceptibles times the density of sources of infection. The pattern of spread following the introduction of a small nucleus of infection (the initial story) into a population of uninfected humans (journalists) and vectors (media outlets) would, if plotted, give an S-shaped curve identical in general form to that shown in Fig. 6.2. It has been suggested that the absence of strong rival stories contributed to the wide coverage given to necrotizing fasciitis. Examination of media output to test this hypothesis has not been done. However, the abrupt ending of radio and TV coverage on 28 May, when an attack by Prime Minister Major on beggars became the top story, merits further investigation.

Fright factors for *E. coli* O157 include its *involuntary* acquisition, e.g. by consuming seemingly safe but microscopically contaminated ready-to-eat cold meats, its *inequitable* distribution (five times commoner in Scotland than England), its ability to cause *irreversible* damage to kidneys and brain, particularly in *small children*, and its ability to cause death in a painful way (Jeremy Bray, MP: 'As the families of too many of my constituents have discovered, dying from *E. coli* is a horrible way to die', *Hansard*, 15 January 1997). As factors determining media interest, these are almost certainly sufficient to explain the persistence of interest long term. However, with the exception of the twentieth death, none of them seemed to play a role in determining the major fluctuations in the number of enquiries made of me after the beginning of the outbreak. These related either to the deliberations and conclusions of the Expert Group or to political events. The first five of the media triggers listed in Department of Health (1997) map well on to these circumstances; thus the alleged concealment of the Swann Report by the Meat Hygiene Service and the Ministry of Agriculture and the Scottish Secretary provide questions of (1) blame, (2) cover-ups, (3) human interest, (4) links with high-profile personalities, and (5) evidence of conflict.

The necrotizing fasciitis and *E. coli* O157 stories differed not only in the media triggers that evoked and drove them, but in the way that they were covered. *E. coli* has always been handled as a serious story and an important issue. The cartoon by High (Fig. 6.5) published in the *Scotsman* (January 1997) typifies this approach. It illustrates the raising of expectations for remedial action, a function that the media sees itself undertaking on behalf of the public—and an obvious response to the media trigger of *many people being exposed* to the risk, even if at low levels. It contrasts sharply with the Banx cartoon (Fig. 6.6) published in the *Independent on Sunday* at the end of the necrotizing fasciitis episode. Not only does this cleverly combine the juxtaposition of this story and the awarding of the contract for the National Lottery, which was announced on the day that media interest in necrotizing fasciitis peaked, but it carries a message about risk—that being attacked by the flesh-eating bug and winning the lottery were equally improbable—while at the same time evoking an atmosphere of black humour. This was also a feature of other media coverage of necrotizing fasciitis, exemplified by the use of Ian Hislop of *Private Eye* (a second choice after Richard Ingrams had declined) for the voice-over of the QED television programme about it made a few weeks after the story had died.

The analysis presented here has not considered the impact of feedback between the media and a frequently used source as a determinant of the properties of this relationship, despite the certainty of its importance. Further work will also be required to establish its impact on media coverage. Such studies would have to take into account the roles that the media regarded myself as playing—for necrotizing faciitis as expert *qua* researcher and for *E. coli* O157 as government-appointed expert—and the roles that I actually played.

Two issues highlighted by the episodes described here are pertinent to risk analysis and risk communication with a far wider relevance than to just infectious disease and food safety. They are clustering, and the trustworthiness of experts. The occurrence of geographical and temporal clusters of

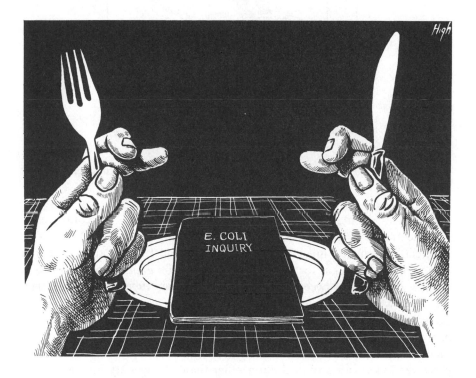

**Fig 6.5**   *The Scotsman*, January 1997 (with permission).

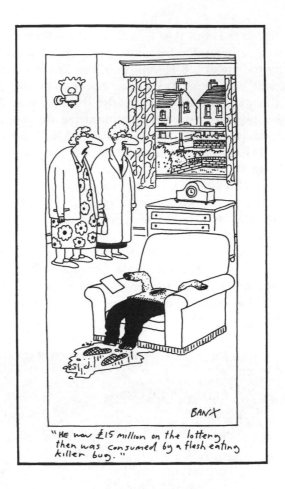

**Fig. 6.6**   *The Independent on Sunday*, May 1994 (with permission).

disease cases, such as leukaemia near nuclear installations, is a controversy. The occurrence of the cluster of cases of necrotising fasciitis at Stroud is no different. It remains unexplained in that biological explanations are still being sought, as well as for the one at Nairn (Upton *et al*. 1995) (four severe invasive infections between October and November 1996 with two deaths), the event which stimulated my initial interest in streptococci. Marris and Langford's (1996) cited ordering of perceived trustworthiness shows why it has been my good fortune to be seen as a doctor (trusted by 75%) rather than a spokesman for the government (trusted by 8%). The absence of perceived links with any institution other than a university may also have been helpful in establishing and maintaining trust. It was embarrassing to be knighted by the *Daily Telegraph* in March 1997 in connection with my obsession with abattoirs, and to be described in other newspapers as foremost, leading, modest, kindly, grave, dogged, determined, dedicated, and white-haired (references available on request)—images redolent of a homogenate of Captain Scott and Santa Claus. While it is objectionable to share the images of both a failure and a myth, it is perhaps comforting to know that for one 'expert' at least, the media retains the positive image of a scientist very similar to that found by Margaret Mead (Mead and Métraux 1957) in her survey of US high school students more than 30 years ago!

## REFERENCES

Cartwright, K., Logan, M., McNulty, C. M., Harrison, S., George, R., Efstratious, A., *et al.* 1995. A cluster of cases of streptococcal necrotizing fasciitis in Gloucestershire. *Epidemiology and Infection*, **115**, 387–97.

Department of Health (1997). *Communicating about risks to public health. Pointers to good practice*. Department of Health, London.

Curran, J., Douglas, A., and Whannel, G. (1980). The political economy of the human-interest story. In *Newspapers and democracy: international essays in a changing medium*, (ed. A. Smith). MIT Press, Cambridge, Mass.

Fishman, M. (1981). Crime waves as ideology. In *The manufacture of news: deviance, social problems and the mass media*, (ed. S. Cohen and J. Young), pp. 98–117. Constable, London.

Galtung, J. and Ruge, M. (1973). Structuring and selecting news. In *The manufacture of news: deviance, social problems and the mass media*, (ed. S. Cohen and J. Young), pp. 52–63. Constable, London.

Hartley, J. (1982). *Understanding news*. Methuen, London.

Haslam, C. and Boyman, A. (ed.) (1994). *Social scientists meet the media*. Routledge, London.

Kitzinger, J. and Reilly, J. (1997). The rise and fall of risk reporting: media coverage of human genetics research. 'False memory syndrome' and 'Mad cow disease'. *European Journal of Communication*, **12**, 319–50.

Lewenstein. B. V. (1995). Science and the media. In *Handbook of science and technology studies*, (ed. S. Jasanoff, G. E. Markle, J. C. Petersen, and T. Pinch). SAGE, Thousand Oaks, California.

Marris, C. and Langford, I. (1996). No cause for alarm. *New Scientist*, 28 September, pp. 36–9.

Mead, M. and Métraux, R. (1957). The image of the scientist among high school students: a pilot study. *Science*, **126**, 384–90.

Nelkin, D. (1989). Journalism and science: the creative tension. In *Health risks and the press: perspectives on media coverage of risk assessment and health*, (ed. M. Moore). The Media Institute, Washington.

Pennington, T. H. (1995). Necrotizing fasciitis: quantitative characteristics of the 1994 British media outbreak. *Journal of Infection*, **30**, 63–5.

Pennington, T. H. (1997). The Pennington Group. Report on the circumstances leading to the 1996 outbreak of infection with *E. coli* O157 in central Scotland, the implications for food safety and the lessons to be learned.

Reilly, J. and Miller, D. (1997). Scaremonger or scapegoat? The role of the media in the emergence of food as a social issue. In *Food, identity and health*, (ed. P. Caplan), pp. 234–51. Routledge, London.

Upton, M., Carter, P. E., Morgan, M., Edwards, G. F., and Pennington, T. H. (1995). Clonal structure of *Streptococcus pyogenes* in northern Scotland. *Epidemiology and Infection*, **115**, 231–41.

# 7 The British Government's handling of risk: some reflections on the BSE/CJD crisis

Robert J. Maxwell
*Formerly Chief Executive, the King's Fund*

## Introduction

As is clear from many of the other contributions to this volume, BSE/CJD has cast a long shadow, not least in its effect on trust in government as a reliable source of information on risk. Here, as elsewhere, the risk communication aspects of the story can only be understood in the context of what was happening in terms of risk identification and assessment. This chapter offers, firstly, a brief summary of what happened and then some reflections on it.

## A summary of events

### BSE in cattle

Bovine Spongiform Encephalopathy (BSE) was first identified in November 1986 by the Ministry of Agriculture, Fisheries and Food (MAFF) Central Laboratory, Weybridge. It belongs to a group of diseases known as Transmissible Spongiform Encephalopathies (TSEs) which affect the brain, leading to confusion, loss of mobility, and ultimately death. There is no effective treatment for BSE and no cure.

The course of the epidemic up to April 1996 is shown in Fig. 7.1, and a chronology of events in Table 7.1. I have summarized the story to mid-1997 more fully elsewhere (Maxwell 1997). Much has already been written about it, and much more will be written in the future. By 31 October 1996 there had been around 164 000 reported cases in Great Britain, around 1700 in Northern Ireland, and a scattering in other countries, mainly in cattle

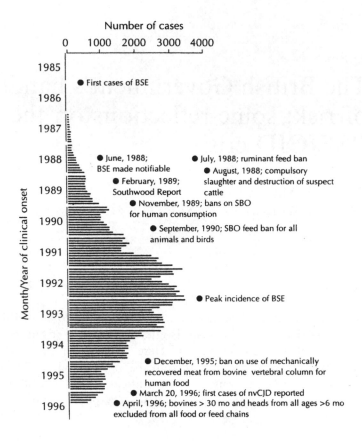

**Fig. 7.1** Confirmed cases of BSE by date of clinical onset, 1986 to May 1996. (From Collee and Bradley (1997).)

imported from the UK. (These figures are likely to be understated, both in Great Britain and outside it, because of under-reporting. Few people, however, would dispute that the epidemic has centred on this country.)

All the evidence points to contaminated feed as the most likely source of the trouble, and specifically to meat and bone meal (MBM) which contained rendered material from sheep and cattle. This was widely used as a cheap source of protein. While much of it may have been harmless enough, some appears to have contained lethal material stemming from the brains and spinal cords of infected animals. In July 1988, following advice from the Southwood Working Party, the feeding of ruminant-derived MBM to cattle was banned by the UK Government. Since the incubation period for BSE in cattle is about 5 years, and since there is probably only limited (mother-to-

**Table 7.1**  Chronology of events

| Date | Event |
| --- | --- |
| November 1986 | BSE first identified by Central Veterinary Laboratory |
| 5 June 1987 | Chief Veterinary Officer (CVO) informs Minister of Agriculture about new disease |
| 15 December 1987 | Initial epidemiological studies completed, which conclude that ruminant-derived meat and bone meal (MBM) was the only viable hypothesis for the cause of BSE |
| 3 March 1988 | Department of Health informed. Expert Advisory Committee recommended |
| 21 April 1988 | Southwood Working Party established. As a result, government indicated it would legislate to make BSE notifiable and to ban ruminant-derived MBM |
| 21 June 1988 | BSE Order 1988 made BSE notifiable |
| July 1988 | Following advice from Southwood, decision announced to introduce slaughter of all affected cattle, and ban on ruminant-derived MBM comes into force |
| 8 August 1988 | Compensation Order introduced. Compensation set at 50% of value for confirmed cases, 100% for negative; both subject to a ceiling |
| February 1989 | Southwood Report received and published, with government's response. Establishment of Tyrrell Committee on research announced (as recommended by Southwood) |
| 10 June 1989 | Tyrrell Report received by government |
| 13 June 1989 | Decision to introduce offals ban announced—not a Southwood recommendation but a government initiative |
| 28 July 1989 | EC ban on export of cattle born before 18 July 1988 and offspring of affected or suspect animals |
| 13 November 1989 | Ban on specified bovine offals (SBO) came into force |
| 9 January 1990 | Tyrrell Report on research and government response to it published |
| 14 February 1990 | Compensation figures changed (see 8 August 1988). Full compensation would be paid, up to a ceiling |
| 1 March 1990 | EC restricts exports of cattle to animals under six months |
| 1 April 1990 | Disease made notifiable to European Commission |
| 3 April 1990 | Spongiform Encephalopathy Committee (SEAC) established under chairmanship of Dr David Tyrrell |
| 9 April 1990 | EC decision to ban export of SBO and other tissues |
| 11 April 1990 | Humberside County Council withdraws British beef from school meals |
| 24 July 1990 | Dr Tyrrell writes publicly to the Chief Medical Officer to say 'any risk as a result of eating beef or beef products is minute. Thus we believe that there is no scientific reason for not eating British beef and that it can be eaten by everyone.' |
| 25 September 1990 | Ban on the use of SBO extended to its inclusion in any animal feed. Export of such feed to other EU member states also banned. (Exports outside the EU banned 10 July 1991.) |
| 15 October 1990 | Farmers required to maintain breeding and movement records |
| 27 June 1994 | Prohibition on the feeding of mammalian protein to ruminants throughout the EU, other than Denmark |
| 1 April 1995 | Compulsory blue staining of SBO |
| 15 August 1995 | The Specified Bovine Offal Order 1995 consolidated and tightened the existing rules for processing SBO |

**Table 7.1**  (*contd*)

| Date | Event |
| --- | --- |
| Autumn 1995 | Spot checks disclose widespread failures to comply with regulations in the handling of SBO in abattoirs (48%) and knackeries and hunt kennels (65%) |
| 28 November 1995 | Acting on advice from SEAC, government announced its decision to stop the use of bovine vertebral column in the manufacture of mechanically-recovered meat. |
| 20 March 1996 | Government announces ten cases of new-style CJD, and their possible link with BSE. Further control measures introduced. Cattle over 30 months must be deboned and trimmings kept out of the food chain |
| 27 March 1996 | EU ban on all UK beef exports, whether to Member States or to other countries |
| 28 March 1996 | Government announces calf slaughter scheme and financial aid for the rendering industry |
| 3 April 1996 | Introduction of 30-month slaughter scheme to ensure that all cattle over 30 months at the time of slaughter do no enter the human or animal food chains |
| 21/22 June 1996 | Florence Summit of the European Council agrees framework of actions required by the UK prior to any lifting of the export ban |
| 29 August 1996 | Professor Anderson of Oxford and his team in collaboration with Wilesmith and others at the Central Veterinary Laboratory publish their analysis of the BSE epidemic in *Nature* (Anderson *et al.* 1996), predicting that the epidemic will virtually die out around 2001 irrespective of further measures |

Source: Ministry of Agriculture, Fisheries and Food (1996).

calf) transmission from animal to animal, one would have expected the epidemic to die out soon after July 1993. In fact, as Fig. 7.1 shows, it had peaked by then but was nowhere near dying out, for two reasons. First, there is considerable variation in the incubation period. Secondly, and more serious in a discussion of risk, some 30 000 calves born after the July 1988 ban later developed the disease (Collee and Bradley 1997). Some of this continuation might be attributable to contamination in the processing plants from lingering traces of feed containing MBM. But the main source is likely to have been various circumventions of the ban, such as use of stocks held by farmers, distributors, and manufacturers. Moreover until September 1990, feed containing specified bovine offals (SBO) could still be used for animals other than cattle, such as pigs and poultry. It seems likely that some farmers continued to use it for cattle, in defiance of the ban.

Nevertheless, incidence began to decline early in 1993. While the epidemic is not yet over, the likelihood is that it will work itself out by around the year 2001 (Anderson *et al.* 1996).

## A risk to human health?

Even when the seriousness of the BSE epidemic was recognized in terms of animal health, most experts maintained that the risk to humans was minimal. As noted in Table 7.1, Dr David Tyrrell, the initial chairman of the Spongiform Encephalopathy Committee (SEAC), wrote publicly to the Chief Medical Officer on 24 July 1990 stating that:

> 'any risk as a result of eating beef or beef products is minute. Thus we believe that there is no scientific reason for not eating British beef and that it can be eaten by everyone'.

Sir Richard Southwood, who had chaired the Working Party on BSE and its implications, took a similar view. Both were influenced by evidence that the TSEs do not readily jump the barrier from one species to another. Scrapie, for example, has been common in sheep in some parts of the world for centuries, but did not appear to have posed a threat to human health. In one important respect, however, Sir Richard was more cautious than Dr Tyrrell. His report recognized that *if his assumption proved wrong*, 'the implications would be extremely serious' (Department of Health and Ministry of Agriculture, Fisheries and Food 1989). Early in 1997, the balance of the evidence suddenly shifted.

## New variant CJD

Creutzfeldt-Jakob Disease (CJD) is the main TSE in man. A classification of human TSEs is shown in Table 7.2. The disease occurs sporadically, virtually throughout the world at the low rate of about one case per two million people each year. It can also be caused by human intervention, for example through the infection of growth hormone derived from human cadaveric pituitary—at one time an accepted treatment for children whose growth was severely retarded. A related disease, called Kuru, was first reported in 1957

**Table 7.2** Ironside's classification of human TSEs

| | |
|---|---|
| Idiopathic | Sporadic CJD |
| Acquired    (Human Source) | Iatrogenic CJD |
| | Kuru |
| (Bovine Source) | new variant CJD |
| Genetic | Familial CJD |
| | Gerstmann-Straussler-Schinker Syndrome (GSS) |
| | Fatal familial insomnia |

Source: Ironside (1998).

in Papua New Guinea. Its cause was in due course shown to be ritualistic cannibalism: the tribe concerned ate their dead relatives as a mark of respect. It occurred mainly in the women and children of the tribe, who ate the less desirable parts including offal. The men ate the prime cuts, which proved less dangerous.

In March 1996 the British government was alerted through SEAC to an article about to be published in *The Lancet* by R. G. Will, himself a member of SEAC, on ten cases of a new variant of CJD, remarkably similar to Kuru in its effects on the brain (Will *et al.* 1996). While there is still no certainty about the derivation of this disease, a number of pointers (e.g. timing, the UK concentration, and the neuropathological profile of the cases) suggest a link with BSE. What Sir Richard Southwood had labelled as an extremely unlikely but gravely serious possibility appeared to have arrived. On Wednesday 20 March, at 3.30 pm Stephen Dorrell, Secretary of State for Health, accordingly announced to the House of Commons that there might be a link between BSE and the new variant of CJD. Accordingly BSE might, after all, pose a threat to human health.

The implications were of course serious—most of all for those who contracted the disease, and for their families. Its symptoms are most distressing in terms of physical and mental deterioration, followed by death. For the present, there was and is no effective treatment. Economically, there were extremely serious implications for British farming, its suppliers, and the meat processing industry. The implications were almost as serious for farming and related industries elsewhere in Europe. Politically too, there was bound to be an impact, especially in terms of Britain's relations with the rest of the European Union.

So much for what has happened—told, I hope, in a way that is neither sensational nor partisan. Now, some points that are relevant to the government's handling of risk.

# Reflections on the case

## The role of MAFF

Until the crisis of March 1996, the main organ of government policy and action over BSE was the Ministry of Agriculture, Fisheries and Food (MAFF). MAFF was responsible both for the welfare of these industries and for food safety. It has come in for criticism for failing in both these roles, on three grounds:

(1) that it was initially slow and complacent in reacting to BSE once the disease and its likely cause had been identified;

(2)  that it was ineffective in its regulatory functions;

(3)  that the devastating impact on farming and food processing could have been lessened.

Taking the first charge (sloth and complacency) first, there was a delay of more than six months between the identification of the disease and the Minister of Agriculture being informed by the Chief Veterinary Officer (CVO) on 5 June 1987. Not until 3 March 1988, nine months later still, was the Department of Health informed, through the Chief Medical Officer (CMO). Only then were the health implications taken seriously in any public sense, with the setting up of the Southwood Working Party.

The first charge merges into the second (ineffectiveness as a regulator). As the story unfolded (Table 7.1 above), increasingly stringent regulations were put in place about the use of specified bovine offals (SBOs) and the slaughter of cattle. However, some of these seem—at least with hindsight—bound to produce perverse results. Setting compensation initially at 50% value for confirmed cases of BSE and 100% for negative cases, created an obvious incentive to under-report BSE. When the July 1988 ban was placed on feeding ruminant-derived MBM to cattle, did no-one consider the likelihood that—since it would still be available for feeding to pigs and poultry—some farmers would flout the new regulation? Turning to the meat processing industry, the spot checks in Autumn 1995 showed widespread failure to comply with the regulations on the handling of SBO. Throughout the period until the crisis of March 1996 one fears that, as the regulations mounted, the gap between theoretical and actual practice widened.

If the picture up until March 1996 is one of practices changing too little, too late, the picture since then seems at times to show the British government being forced to overreact and going way beyond the scientific evidence in some of the culls imposed. We will return later to the European dimensions of the story.

When something has gone very badly wrong—as it clearly has with over 30 human deaths so far, millions of cattle slaughtered, and a mass of rendered carcasses still to be disposed of—it is tempting to put the blame on individuals or particular institutions such as MAFF. And MAFF does not come well out of the story. But if we leave it at that, we learn little. One relevant factor is that the weight of independent scientific opinion, reflected by Dr David Tyrrell, Sir Richard Southwood and others, was strongly of the view that the risk posed to human health by BSE was minimal. Properly stated, scientific opinion would never have said that there was *no* risk, but leading scientists came close. As late as December 1995, the Secretary of State for Health said that it was 'inconceivable' that CJD could be caused by BSE. He was tempting the Gods, but he was not far away from the prevailing scientific opinion of the time. We need to learn from that: the experts can be wrong, and everyone involved ought to be meticulous about not confusing probabilities and hopes with certainties.

A second influence on MAFF, for which most of us must take some share of the blame, was the assumption that the more intensive the methods used in British farming, the greater its efficiency. We grew up assuming that continental European farming was hopelessly outdated. This is another point to which we shall return. For the present I am simply noting that while MAFF may be a convenient scapegoat, its attitudes were partly shaped by majority opinion—not only in the farming and food industries, but more broadly.

Thirdly, it is clearly a mistake to have given MAFF responsibility for food safety as well as for the promotion of agriculture and fisheries. The economic pressures are for maximum production and cheap food. Food safety pulls in a quite different direction: toward high standards and minimum risks, even at the price of extra fuss and higher costs. Putting the two together in one government department means handling the tensions between them within the fastnesses of the ministry and hiding the conflicts. A result is that food safety received (not only in this instance) less than its due. As is clear throughout this volume, a key issue is trust. Now that something has gone so badly wrong, the public will not trust MAFF again.

## The interplay of science, policy and politics

In some ways, the BSE story provides an object lesson in how government can draw upon expert scientific advice in a way that everybody (including commentators and the public) can understand and respect. From the Southwood Working Party, through the Tyrrell Committee to SEAC, the scientific committees have a good record of absorbing and explaining the evidence in a complex and changing field. They were at times seriously wrong, but their views were reasonable at that point. Moreover, government listened and did not try to influence or censor their advice. As one of the key scientists put it to me:

'The Cabinet truly was motivated to understand. We were put under no pressure to manipulate anything and, since the crisis broke, they have published everything that we have said.'

However, two key features were not so satisfactory: nor are they unique to this case. One, amounting almost to a collusion between scientific orthodoxy and the government, is the policy assumption that the orthodox view of the time must be right. The other is the handling of risk.

Taking the first of these, the Tyrrell Committee was set up in January 1990 to promote research and to monitor BSE. However, little research followed. At this stage, as we have seen, BSE was taken to be an agricultural problem and the leisurely pace was set by the vets in MAFF. What research funding there was went to scientists who themselves subscribed to the orthodox view that BSE posed no threat to man. Despite Southwood's recognition of the implications should this assumption prove wrong, little if any research was promoted to pursue the alternative hypothesis. When there is a small chance that a deadly risk exists, then potentially the most valuable research may be that which takes the non-orthodox view that the risk is real. Instead, anyone who took this line was likely to be branded a scaremonger, not to be taken seriously.

The joint report of the House of Commons Agriculture and Health Committees (1996) records interesting exchanges between MPs, the CMO, the CVO, Professor Pattison of SEAC, Dr Stephen Dealler, and Professor Lang on risk and its handling. In essence, Mr Meldrum, the CVO, took the line that MAFF had all along taken an ultra-precautionary route in BSE policy, acting as though the worst might happen. The CMO pointed out that the risk of contracting CJD appeared to be very low, but that the public perception of the risk was higher than the science said it was. Professor Lang —largely supported by Dr Dealler—took the view that 'BSE has provided an object lesson in how not to manage risk.'

Some points made by Douglas and Wildavsky (1982) in the context of environmental risks are relevant here. The key terms in the debate over risk and technology are, they suggest, risk and acceptability. Calculating the probability of danger (i.e. the risk) concentrates on what is physically 'out there' in man's intervention in the natural world. What is *acceptable* depends on the uncertainty that is 'in here', within a person's mind. Going from 'out there' to 'in here' requires a connection between the dangers of technology and people's perceptions of them. Consequently, it is never enough to assume that the science of risk is only about objective, external danger. It is also about attitudes of mind. Throughout the BSE story—at least until very recently—those in authority in Britain (in government and in science) tended to be quite robust in their perception of the acceptability of a low risk of danger. They have found it difficult to understand those for whom such a risk, even though low, is unacceptable.

## The European dimension

One of the worst parts of the handling of the BSE crisis by the British government was the European dimension, and we are not out of the wood yet. There is a legacy both of damaged relations with our European partners and of policies that have little to recommend them. It also seems inevitable that whatever lessons are learnt from the BSE affair will have to be applicable not only within Britain but at the European level.

When Stephen Dorrell and Douglas Hogg made their statements to the House of Commons on 20 March 1996, cattle prices and beef consumption at once began to fall, not only in Britain but across Europe. A European crisis was in train. Allegedly Franz Fischler, the Agriculture Commissioner, had only half an hour's warning of the announcement. If that is true, it seems downright silly. Britain would need all the goodwill and cooperation it could muster from other European governments and from Brussels. On 27 March, following unilateral bans by individual governments on British beef exports, the European Commission imposed a collective ban. At this point the British government quickly started to play domestic politics by blaming Brussels. One can see how tempting that must have been, given the strong 'anti-Europe' strand in the Conservative Party, and indeed across the spectrum of British public opinion. But it was not at all clever to stir up British public opinion to bolster a head-on confrontation with Brussels and a policy of non-cooperation in routine business. What the Commission had done was an inevitable expression of the views of all the other parties to the Union. Non-cooperation caused maximum affront at the most sensitive time, with absolutely no justification except in terms of British domestic politics.

Another, quite different, concern is about the processes and outcomes of policy formulation at the European level. Naturally enough, the EU has its own expert committees, policy processes, and methods of negotiating consensus. In this particular case, a result was the Florence Agreement of June 1996 which accepted a framework proposed by the Commission for step-by-step relaxations of the ban. There was no guarantee that, if followed, this would actually result in the lifting of the ban, and little justification for the agreed cull of 140 000 cattle. What is more, details of the culls, e.g. the differentiation by birth cohorts, are difficult to implement and monitor. Far more than 140 000 cattle have already been culled since the Florence Agreement, but it is questionable whether the details have been complied with. The principal elements of the ban remained in force. All in all, the challenges of relating science, policy, and action at the European level are even greater than those within the UK.

## Farming and food policy

As I have put it elsewhere,

> 'Something has gone seriously wrong with our food policy, and one can see why. As consumers we want cheap food. Indeed compared with the

Germans and the Dutch we seem bent on food bargains, ahead of concerns about quality. We appear to have come to assume that anything on sale is safe. By now, we ought to know better. *Salmonella* in eggs (1988), *Listeria* in soft cheese (1990), toxin in apple juice (1993), traces of phthalates in baby food (1996), *E. coli* in beef (1996) are all serious instances of food dangers, quite apart from BSE'.

(Maxwell 1997)

Food is among the most important influences on human health. It is time for us all, the broader public, to take a serious interest in the quality of our food and therefore in the methods by which it is produced. It is time for public opinion and government to insist that food policy is more risk-averse, and that incentives are in place to encourage safer farming. As a result, our food will cost us more. As Professor Hugh Pennington has said in launching his report on *E. coli*, the public will have to pay 'significantly more' to cover the costs of safer methods—perhaps between 10 and 50% more (*The Sunday Times*, 30 March 1997).

# Closing reflections

So far, over 30 people have died a particularly unpleasant and early death from new variant CJD. Their only recklessness was to trust all those who told them that eating British beef was safe. It is still much too early to predict the final scale of the tragedy. For example, there is a dawning recognition of the potential danger of transmission through contaminated blood. Even if, by extraordinarily good luck, there were to be no further deaths, we should resolve to learn from this tragic—and in some ways sordid—story. In the context of public health and risk communication, I shall confine myself to four lessons:

- **Opt for safer food at higher cost**. We did not have to turn ruminants into unwitting cannibals in the first place. Once the regulations began to be tightened there seems to have been a widespread willingness in the animal feed, farming, and meat processing industries to continue cutting corners rather than take the trouble to comply. Remember also all those who have died from *E. coli* and other failures in food safety. The next major threat to public health will doubtless take a different form, but future threats there will be. Let us therefore be ready—not only in government but throughout the food chain—to see that risks are not taken recklessly (and at times cynically) with human lives.

- **Put in place arrangements to enable issues about risk to be publicly articulated and understood.** This means that scientific advice must be authoritative and independent, as it has been in SEAC. However, it also means acknowledging Douglas and Wildavsky's analysis —the need to judge not only the risk physically 'out there' but also the acceptability of that risk 'in here'. The main reason, I suggest, for MAFF's inadequacies as a food safety watchdog was that its personnel saw their role primarily as being about political, economic, and practical trade-offs. Like many others, they were prepared to run a small risk that they might be wrong. We are entitled not only to a different level of protection—a watchdog with teeth—but to public articulation of debate.

- **Resist jumping to the conclusion that what one would like to believe is true.** For nearly ten years, most experts thought that the risk that BSE would harm human beings was negligible. Civil servants, politicians, the public, all wanted to believe that. The current pressure is to be reassured that the worst is now past and that the number of human deaths will remain relatively low. In both cases, the scientists need to explain uncertainty, and resolutely decline to be drawn into statements that offer false reassurance. There is all the difference in the world, in terms of scientific integrity, between the forecast by Anderson *et al.* (1996) of decline in BSE incidence, where the reasoning behind the forecast is carefully explained, and any statement at the moment about the ultimate range of numbers of new-style CJD. Because of uncertainties—for example over whether there will be infection via contaminated blood—it is simply too early to say. For the moment that is the message by which the scientists must stand and which the rest of us must accept— however uncomfortable that may be.

- **Act on the lessons learned, not only nationally, but at the European level.** Food safety is a public health issue in terms of the Treaty of Europe, and food is an international commodity. It seems certain that the EU will be more risk-averse in food policy than Britain has been, because several European nations (including Germany and Holland) have already shown themselves not to be risk takers in this field. But that gives no guarantee that the arrangements for handling food safety in Brussels— and for dealing with crises when they occur—will be efficient and effective. The effort that we put in now at the European level must be not only about reducing the damage done to British interests by the whole affair, but about making food safe for the future.

## REFERENCES

Anderson, R. M., Donnelly, C. A., Ferguson, N. M., Woolhouse, M. E. J., *et al.* (1996). Transmission dynamics and epidemiology of BSE in British cattle. *Nature*, **382**, 779–88 .

Collee, J. G. and Bradley, R. (1997). BSE: a decade on—part 2. *The Lancet*, **349**, 718.

Department of Health and Ministry of Agriculture, Fisheries and Food (1989). *Report of the working party on bovine spongiform encephalopathy (the Southwood report)*, Paragraph 9.2, ISBN 15197 4059. Department of Health and Ministry of Agriculture, Fisheries and Food, London.

Douglas, M. and Wildavsky, A. (1982). *Risk and culture*. University of California Press, Berkeley.

House of Commons Agriculture and Heath Committees (1996). *BSE and CJD: recent developments*, HC-331. HMSO, London.

Ironside, J. W. (1998). Creutzfeldt-Jakob disease—the story so far. *Proceedings of the Royal College of Physicians of Edinburgh*, **28**, 143.

Ministry of Agriculture, Fisheries and Food (1996). In *House of Commons Agriculture and Health Committees' joint reports: BSE and CJD: recent developments* (1996) and *BSE in Great Britain: a progress report* (November 1996). Ministry of Agriculture, Fisheries and Food, London.

Maxwell, R. J. (1997). *An unplayable hand? BSE, CJD and British Government*. King's Fund, London.

Will, R. G., Ironside, J. W., Zeidler, M., *et al.* (1996). A new variant of Creutzfeldt-Jakob disease in the UK. *The Lancet*, **347**, 921–7.

# 8 Experiences in risk communication

Ronan A. Lyons and Dorothy Wright

*Consultant/Senior Lecturer in Public Health Medicine, Welsh Combined Centres for Public Health* and *Deputy Director of Public Health and CCDC, Iechyd Morgannwg Health*

## Introduction

Over the past five years, consultants from the Welsh Combined Centres for Public Health and the Department of Public Health of Iechyd Morgannwg Health have been involved with a considerable number of environmental issues resulting in public anxiety over potential health effects, and have had experience of both successful and unsuccessful risk communication practices. We have been involved with health scares over suspected leukaemia clustering around a chemical plant, neurological disorders in bathers at a particular beach, opencast mining and asthma, the Sea Empress oil spill, a chemical incident involving fatalities and large numbers of affected people, and asbestos dust in flats, to name some of the more high-profile cases.

This chapter draws on six specific episodes. For each there follows a brief description of the incident, our involvement in risk communication, and the lessons learnt.

## The cases

### Suspected leukaemia clustering around a chemical plant

Since the 1980s concern had been expressed by local people that the incidence of cancer in the Sandfields area of Port Talbot and around the BP Chemical site at Baglan Bay was higher than normal, and particularly so for leukaemia and lymphoma in children and young adults. The situation was investigated by the Welsh Cancer Registry in 1989 and no excess cancer was detected. However, because of ongoing local concerns the matter was referred to the Small Areas Health Statistics Unit (SAHSU ) at the London School of Hygiene and Tropical Medicine by the Welsh Office.

Just before its report was due to be published, a television company became interested in the topic and started its own investigation. We learnt of the situation through the headmaster of the local school which had been visited by the media. Following discussions with the television company it became clear that they were convinced they had uncovered an excess of cancer in the area and were going to broadcast a programme before the SAHSU report was to be released.

We decided to check the accuracy of the company's findings by carrying out our own investigation, since we could not gain access to the SAHSU report as it had not been cleared by the Departments of Health. Our investigation involved checking the details of all cases of leukaemia and lymphoma in the area over a 25-year period, which revealed several errors in coding and incorrect addresses at the time of diagnosis. The net result was that the alleged cluster of leukaemia did not exist.

Two days before the programme was due to be broadcast we called a press conference and released our results. There was widespread television, radio, and press coverage and the proposed documentary was never screened. The majority of local people were relieved that the incidence of cancer in the area, and in past and present pupils of the school, was within normal limits, although the parents of the children who had died from leukaemia were unhappy that an explanation for their children's deaths had not been found. Our report (Lyons *et al.* 1995) and the SAHSU report (Sans *et al.* 1995) were later published in the scientific press, both confirming that rates of leukaemia around the plant were within normal limits.

## Neurological disorders in bathers at Oxwich Bay

In November 1994 two young people were reported in the media as having developed paralysis following bathing at a local beach. The beach was a well-known beauty spot with an estimated 100 000 visitors per year. Viruses were thought to be a possible cause of the illnesses, but none had been identified. Over the next few days six people reported a variety of illnesses, predominantly neurological disorders, which they associated with visiting the beach.

The local media focused on the environmental issues surrounding these cases, and a Senior Environmental Health Officer, who had a good relationship with the media, initially contained the speculation.

However, when a newspaper claimed that the three agencies, namely the National Rivers Authority, Welsh Water, and the City Council, with power to investigate the problem, had failed to do so, the National Rivers Authority independently announced to the press that there was to be an emergency meeting of all agencies involved. This announcement was made on Saturday and by Monday the national press had been galvanized into action with wide publicity of the story. At the same time there were now suggestions that the cause of the illnesses could be due to algae or chemicals from maritime wrecks. The problem was not going to go away!

The Consultant in Communicable Disease Control (CCDC) attended the emergency meeting. As a result, the issue was refocused away from the environmental issues to the health aspects, and from then on it became a health-led investigation with support from other agencies.

Anyone who believed that they had an illness connected with having been on the beach or in the sea were invited to contact the CCDC. Twenty-one people reported illnesses, and investigations covering epidemiological, clinical, microbiological, and environmental aspects were carried out into each case. The investigations failed to find a link between reported illnesses, or between illnesses and the beach (Wright 1995). At a personal level, only one individual continued to be dissatisfied with the outcome, but some of the local population are wary and do not bathe there anymore!

During the course of the investigation it became clear that one particular journalist was avidly pursuing the story, often when there was nothing new to report, and despite the evidence to the contrary, was determined to demonstrate an underlying scandal and 'cover up'. The perceived health risk to those affected needed to be recognized and their concerns acknowledged, but the investigation was hampered at an early stage when issues of litigation and compensation were raised, which sometimes made the interpretation of symptoms difficult.

While the stance of the regulatory authorities in denying an association between bathing at the beach and subsequent illness was later confirmed by the investigation, this was initially seen by many as protecting the tourist trade (privatization) and defending their own failure to undertake viral sampling (requested by pressure groups), when their prime responsibility should have been to protect the public health and environment.

## Opencast mining and asthma

Concerns about the potential health effects of opencast mining in the area were heightened following the publication of a paper in the *British Medical Journal* by a local general practitioner (Temple and Sykes 1992), demonstrating a two-fold increase in asthma following the opening of an adjacent mine.

We were approached by the local county council to comment on the potential for health effects following a planning application for a second mine in the vicinity. Our review of the evidence indicated that there was insufficient evidence on which to base an opinion, one way or the other, and recommended that further research be carried out. Following widespread consultation on the issues, involving local councillors, local authority officers, concerned parents and teachers, it was decided to proceed with a study into the effects of pollutants from all sources on children's respiratory health. The study was jointly funded by West Glamorgan Health Authority, West Glamorgan County Council, Swansea City Council, Neath Borough Council, and Celtic Energy (previously known as British Coal Opencast). The parents of all children aged 8–10 were approached in the three areas to be studied, and 99% agreed to their children's involvement.

The results of the study were made public at a press conference, an explanation and copies having been circulated to participating schools and funding bodies the day before (Lyons *et al.* 1997). The study revealed that there was an effect of dust on children's respiratory function at the site nearest the mine, that the effect was small, that technology had not evolved to the point of being able to fingerprint the exact source of the dust responsible for the health effect, and that most of the dust came from outside the immediate area. The report was warmly received by local people and elected members, despite the fact that it was not possible to answer all the questions.

## Sea Empress oil spill

In February 1996 the Sea Empress oil tanker ran aground at Milford Haven, Pembrokeshire, spilling 72 000 tons of oil which contaminated over 200 km of some of the most beautiful coastline in Britain. The local health authority was not invited to the initial emergency meeting as the major issues were felt to be environmental. However, in the week following the spill many people living along the coastline complained of being unwell.

The health authority sought the advice of the Welsh Combined Centres for Public Health on appropriate studies to evaluate the impact of the oil spill on the health of the local population. Subsequently, the health authority commissioned a study into the acute physical and psychological impact of the oil spill. The study involved a comparison of symptoms and illness in random samples of 1000 residents in the most exposed areas and 1000 controls selected from unexposed areas. A report into the findings of the study was presented to the health authority board, the public, and the media in December (Lyons *et al.* 1996). This report indicated that there had been a substantial increase in physical and psychological problems following the oil spill. The report was warmly welcomed by local people and the member of parliament.

Because of continued community concerns and the findings of the study, Dyfed Powys Health Authority commissioned a follow-up study into people's health one year after the oil spill. This study involved not only all those who had participated in the earlier study, but also included their children and elderly people who had not been previously involved. The follow-up study was presented to the health authority in the beginning of 1998 (Lyons *et al.* 1998). It revealed that while there was still a substantial psychological impact, there was no evidence of any increase in serious physical illness. The Health Authority accepted the report's recommendation to continuously monitor serious illness in the exposed population so as to be able to address any public anxieties which might arise in the future.

## Fatal chemical incident at Crymlyn Burrows

In October 1996 two local authority workmen collapsed and died while emptying a sewer pumping station where a pump had been malfunctioning for some weeks. Rescue workers who recovered the bodies and the ambulancemen who took the victims to the mortuary complained of a sharp smell of chemicals. Subsequently, many people attending the site became ill and were referred to the accident and emergency unit with a variety of problems. Seventeen people were admitted to hospital.

Two chemicals, freon II and methylstyrene, were identified in the samples taken from the pumping station and the disposal vehicle used by the workmen. Members of our department of public health worked closely with colleagues in the accident and emergency department, the local authority, and emergency services in managing and investigating the incident. Work continued for several days around the sewer to repair the malfunctioning pump. Full breathing apparatus was used by people working on the site.

The pumping station was within 30 m of a street of houses. Residents had been distressed at the death of the two local men and were obviously concerned when they observed workers in full protective clothing operating so close to their homes. Media coverage was also high.

Recognizing that the scale and the severity of this incident was likely to have an impact on the residents, public health doctors visited each household and carried out a risk assessment, including taking biological samples. Analysis revealed low levels of freon II in the blood of several residents. All residents were advised of their results and a follow-up evaluation was carried out six months later.

The findings and their implications were explained to the residents in their own homes which allowed for an open and frank discussion. The actions of the department in quickly recognizing and investigating the risk to residents was much appreciated by them. The relationship which had developed between the department and residents was of value when problems with the sewer system, relating to the incident, re-emerged.

A report of the incident was provided to the Health Authority (Wright 1997).

## Asbestos dusts in local authority housing

The cleaning of vent grilles in a local-authority-owned flat complex revealed a small amount of asbestos dust (amosite) in the vent shaft. Asbestos-lagged pipes had been removed three years earlier and the remaining rubble boarded over. Samples taken after the clearance were clear of asbestos.

In light of the new findings, the local authority Environmental Health Department took air samples from the flats. Traces of asbestos, albeit well within the exposure limits, were found in eight out of 34 flats. Arrangements were made for dust removal by a specialist contractor and a programme of air testing was instigated. The Council sent a letter to each of the tenants explaining the position and the action being taken. Meetings were held with officers of the Tenants Association and the tenants themselves. A newsletter was also produced.

The media became very interested in the situation, not least when it was revealed that an elderly tenant had died four years previously from mesothelioma, a tumour usually related to asbestos exposure. Anxiety was high among tenants and there were calls for mass X-ray screening. Members of our department assessed the health risks to the residents.

At a meeting with representatives of the tenants, the risks associated with asbestos at the levels found in the flats, the nature of the illness caused by asbestos, and the risks and benefits of X-ray screening were explained and discussed by public health doctors. The tenants were reassured and accepted that as the additional risks involved with the exposure were so small, X-ray screening may do more harm than good.

# Reflections on health scares and responses to them

Why some health concerns become health scares is often a matter of chance and seems to depend on the characteristics of the individuals concerned, competing stories in the media, and risk communication practices of public health doctors and other individuals. Many concerns are brought to our notice each year which have the potential to become health scares, but for a variety of reasons do not attract media attention.

We feel that there are similarities now between public anxiety relating to environmental health scares and the situation 10 years ago with meningitis. Then, news of a case of meningitis tended to attract widespread media coverage which often exaggerated the risks of death and the likelihood of spread to other members of the community. However, with effective risk communication strategies involving the provision of information on risk, what to look out for and what to do if a problem arises, readily available leaflets, more active intervention (chemoprophylaxis and vaccination), and media management, cases of meningitis no longer result in public hysteria.

The difference with environmental health cases is that the perceived threat is usually posed by an identifiable group or industry rather than by chance, the risks are often not well characterized or are unknown, credible information is not readily available, and effective interventions to reduce the threat in the short term are either impossible or very difficult to implement. In such circumstances it can be very difficult to allay public anxieties.

When a health concern is brought to our attention several aspects need careful consideration before a response can be made:

Is the concern biologically plausible?

Is there any evidence of hazard in the literature?

If the concern does not appear to be well founded, will responding to it create additional media attention and result in a health scare?

If the health concern does appear to be biologically plausible and substantive, how best should we respond?

- by an explanation of what is known and a risk assessment?

- by acknowledgement of uncertainty?

- by the utility or otherwise of a more detailed health and environmental assessment?

If the concern is likely to become a scare anyway, a response is required, but exactly how, where, when, and to whom need careful thought.

Deciding whether or not to investigate an allegation also means considering how much it is going to cost and where the money will come from. More often than not much of the cost has to come from the general health authority budget and therefore be taken from direct patient care. The question of relative benefits needs to be considered. Diverting money from a budget primarily intended to provide health services for the ill to investigate health scares, many of which turn out to be false, may not be in the best interest of the community.

In our experience the things we have found to be helpful in risk communication with the general public are as follows:

1. A clear statement that, as public health physicians, our aim is to protect and promote the health of the public .

2. A clear statement that we are independent of regulatory authorities and industry.

3. A policy of openness and honesty about what is known about specific health risks and what is not known.

4.  Opportunities to meet with concerned individuals and groups to discuss issues rather than relying too much on formal correspondence.

5.  Involving community groups in study aims and design where possible, when any extended monitoring or research is required to quantify risk.

6.  The importance of early involvement of public health departments with other agencies in chemical and major incidents to allow health issues to be considered at the earliest stage.

7.  Rapid access to toxicological and environmental databases to provide an evidence-based background.

8.  Commitment by health authorities to the importance of good risk communications and an understanding of the amount of resource needed to offset and deal with crises.

Being accepted by the community as credible, independent assessors of environmental health issues is an essential prerequisite to effective risk communication. Living within the communities one serves is also helpful in this regard, as there is a sense of a sharing of problems and experiences. While one cannot predict the outcome of any investigation in advance, having experience of both negative and positive findings is also valuable. We believe that having substantiated community fears of environmental health effects in some instances but not in others has boosted our credibility in this area.

We are not seen as a body perceived to be involved in 'white-washes' or cover-ups, nor one which is alarmist, but one which will carry out a thorough and independent assessment of environmental health issues.

The things which we have found to be *unhelpful* in communicating risks to the public are as follows:

1.  Responding by a reassurance of 'no health risk' based on absence of evidence. Denials and reassurances alone are usually insufficient to resolve many issues. Even when evidence is sound, there should be an awareness of possible underlying agendas.

2.  Conflicting advice eminating from different agencies. Where multiple agencies are involved a single, agreed spokesperson is preferable. However, it is important to guard against the danger of being perceived as being influenced by 'vested interests'.

3.  Difficulty in accessing previous research data about health risks.

4.  The temptation to use inadequate studies which only lead to a long-term loss of public credibility.

5.  In national health scares, being contacted by a journalist before the opportunity to peruse information from the Health Department's cascade system.

## REFERENCES

Lyons, R. A., Monaghan, S. P., Heaven, M., Littlepage, B. N. C., Vincent, T. J., and Draper, G. J. (1995). Incidence of leukaemia and lymphoma in young people in the vicinity of the petrochemical plant at Baglan Bay, South Wales, 1974 to 1991. *Occupational and Environmental Medicine*, **52**, 225–8.

Lyons, R. A., Temple, M., Evans, D., and Palmer, S. (1996). *Report to Dyfed Powys Health Authority on the acute effects of the Sea Empress oil spill on the health of the South Pembrokeshire population*. Welsh Combined Centres for Public Health, School of Postgraduate Studies in Medicine and Health Care, Swansea.

Lyons, R. A., Fielder, H., Heaven, M., Morgan, H., Govier, P., Erikson, A., *et al.* (1997). *Report on the acute effects of air pollution on the respiratory health of children in West Glamorgan*. Welsh Combined Centres for Public Health, School of Postgraduate Studies in Medicine and Health Care, Swansea.

Lyons, R. A., Temple, M., Evans, D., and Palmer, S. (1998). *Report to Dyfed Powys Health Authority on the one year follow-up study into potential health effects of the Sea Empress oil spill on the population of South Pembrokeshire*. Welsh Combined Centres for Public Health, School of Postgraduate Studies in Medicine and Health Care, Swansea.

Sans, S., Elliott, P., Kleinschmidt, I., Shaddick, G., Pattenden, S., Grundy, C., *et al.* (1995). Cancer incidence and mortality near the Baglan Bay petrochemical works, South Wales. *Occupational and Environmental Medicine*, **52**, 217–24.

Temple, J. M. F. and Sykes, A. M. (1992). Asthma and opencast mining. *British Medical Journal*, **305**, 396–7.

Wright, D. (1995). *Oxwich Bay investigation*. West Glamorgan Health Authority, Swansea.

Wright, D. (1997). *Chemical incident at Crymlyn Burrows*. Iechyd Morgannwg Health Authority, Swansea.

# 9 Benchmarking in government: case studies and principles

Tony Taig
*Risk Solutions, AEA Technology plc*

## Introduction

This chapter is based on a project sponsored by a number of government departments and agencies and carried out under contract by AEA Technology during 1997–98 (Health and Safety Executive 1998). Its aims were:

- to evaluate government experience and lessons learned
- to develop some simple principles of good practice
- to develop guidance for government to help improve practice in communicating about risks and the measures for their control.

From the outset, the study set out to consider communication as a two-way issue, involving listening, understanding, and engagement of the public in the regulatory process, as well as the effective dissemination of information and advice. The principal project activity was a series of case studies, working with departments and agencies to explore and evaluate recent experiences and identify lessons. Four major case studies covered:

- drink-driving
- infant feeding, including several specific issues
- land use planning around hazardous installations
- organophosphate use in agriculture.

The project also involved a series of workshops, a literature survey, and a trawl of industrial and commercial experience including a collection of case histories from a well-known public relations and communications consultancy. A fifth case study within government assembled anecdotes on different experiences in crisis communication.

This chapter describes briefly the four case studies listed above, and introduces four principles for good practice in risk communication derived from them and from the other sources drawn on. Some observations on government performance are offered, and the conclusions and recommendations for practice summarized. Some wider observations on risk communication are presented in Chapter 17.

# The case studies

## Drink-driving

Social attitudes to drink-driving have changed radically in the UK over the past two decades, though even today some 500 people are killed in drink-related accidents on the UK roads each year This case study examined the history of the approach adopted by the (then) UK Department of Transport (DoT) since the mid-1970s, in terms of both communication and regulation/enforcement.

A landmark in the fight against drink-driving was a major independent review, the 'Blennerhasset Report' (Department of the Environment 1976). This report recognized that regulation and enforcement activities alone were not sufficient to alter public behaviour. Sustained commitment to education and communication, to win hearts and minds to the importance of the issue, was recommended.

Since that time, a major publicity campaign has been waged by the DoT, in conjunction with education, enforcement, and new, tougher regulations. Virtually everybody in the UK is familiar with the major TV advertizing campaigns mounted against drink-driving most Christmases in the past 20 years.

A very notable feature of the communication campaigns is their strong management and planning across all the various agencies involved—DoT, the police and emergency services, advertising experts, 'stakeholder' organizations, and opinion researchers. Enforcement activity is carefully planned to reinforce the messages put out in the communications campaigns. Local government, motoring organizations, and alcoholic drink manufacturers (to name but a few) are mobilized to set up parallel initiatives to get across and reinforce the messages. Detailed analysis of accident statistics is used to identify the key target audiences, and thorough opinion research is carried out before and after each campaign to test its effectiveness.

Viewed solely as a series of advertising campaigns, the DoT initiatives have been resoundingly successful. For example, the 'Dave' campaign of Christmas 1995 was reported by *Marketing Magazine* as achieving public recognition running at 91% in January and 89% six months later. The only

UK campaign to beat this performance was the BT 'good to talk' campaign, which spent £90 million compared with the DoT's £2 million. (The 'Dave' campaign focused on young, 'at risk' drivers. It aimed to maximize social awareness of the problem and maintain social pressure on potential offenders by showing a mother spoon-feeding a young man, mentally and physically disabled in a crash after his mates had urged 'just one more' on him.)

Viewed as part of the overall campaign against drink-driving, the communications initiatives have also been highly effective. Some key statistics indicate the improvements in drink-driving behaviour and attitudes in the UK between 1985 and 1995:

- drink-driving fatalities have dropped from 1040 in 1985 to around 540 in 1995
- the failure rate of breath tests has dropped from 28.1% (out of 45 000 tests) to 6.3% (out of 119 000 tests) over the same period
- significant shifts in drink-driving attitudes are indicated by the figures in Table 9.1 from research carried out for DoT by the Central Office of Information:

It is impossible to say how much of the change is attributable to the DoT campaigns and how much to legislation, enforcement, and other initiatives. But road safety experts inside and outside government agree that, at the very least, the communication campaigns have created a climate in which there is greater social acceptance of tougher legislation and enforcement. There is probably a symbiosis—legislation cannot succeed without effective communication, and communication cannot succeed without effective legislation and enforcement.

**Table 9.1** Changes in attitudes and behaviour claimed by people questioned about drink-driving in 1979 and 1995

| Behaviour/attitude | Percentage claiming behaviour | |
| --- | --- | --- |
| | 1979 | 1995 |
| Drinking after driving at least once in the last week | 51 | 25 |
| Drinking 6+ units and then driving | 15 | 4 |
| Leaving the car at home when going drinking | 54 | 75 |
| Avoiding risk and arranging for someone else to drive | 48 | 61 |
| It's hard to avoid drinking and driving in the social context | 61 | 25 |
| Knowing having to drive spoils the evening | 64 | 48 |

Source: Central Office of Information (Health & Safety Executive 1998).

This case study highlights the importance of communication for effective implementation of mandatory risk control measures. It also demonstrates the vital importance of the management process for coordinating the agencies and messages involved, and the importance of understanding the audience and its attitudes and opinions—using both 'hard' accident statistics to identify who needs to be reached, and 'soft' opinion research to understand what is likely to be effective in altering its behaviour.

## Infant feeding

This case study examined a series of highly publicized incidents relating to infant feeding in the UK in 1996 and 1997. Risk associated with infant formula—or for that matter with breast milk—is a particularly emotive topic, because of the importance of good nutrition in the early months of life and the effective lack of alternatives to infant formula, once a decision to feed by bottle has been made.

### Phthalates

The first incident involved a health scare over phthalates (a group of chemicals widely present in plastics, such as PVC) in infant formula in the early summer of 1996. The scare related to the possibility of effects of these contaminants on reproductive health in particular, following the discovery in new, sensitive surveillance tests carried out for MAFF (the Ministry of Agriculture, Fisheries and Foods), of above the recommended tolerable levels.

Given the large safety margins built into the defined tolerable levels in foods and the absence of any particular reason to suspect that any one brand was worse than any other, the government advised people not to change their feeding regime (the risks of poor nutrition were considered to outweigh any risk associated with the contaminants), and refused to publish the names of the brands used in the surveillance tests.

The government response was widely perceived as patronizing—dismissive of the risk and of people's concerns about the issue. It provided little help in understanding the nature of the risk, putting the issue in perspective and outlining the pros and cons of the different choices parents might make in response to the news. A particular problem was that the full information about the issue had not been disseminated to medical professionals, so that people were unable to get further information and advice from their local GPs, health visitors, and midwives. Jonathan Porritt wrote in the *Daily Telegraph*:

> '... the Department of Health sent shivers down our spines by declaring that it 'has seen the research papers and there is no cause for alarm'—shades

of Corporal Jones in Dad's Army, who would send everyone into a blue funk with his repeated bellows of 'Don't panic!'.

The end result was a widespread panic reaction, with an unknown but considerable number of parents prematurely weaning infants from formula onto cow's milk, and a strong adverse media and public reaction.

## Phytoestrogens

The next episode considered here followed shortly after the phthalate scare, and involved the high level of phytoestrogens (plant chemicals which in large doses have been shown to be able to affect reproductive health in animals) in some soya-based brands of infant formula. Such formula is used by parents whose children are allergic to other formulations, or who choose soya-based formula through preference of a vegetarian diet.

Again, the government judged the risk to be small, and advised parents not to switch feeding regimes without consulting their doctors or health advisers. But, following the phthalates experience, much more effort was made to communicate proactively, with an advance cascade of information to medical professionals, a press release, and a series of briefings to press and medical professional groups. The media and public response was much more muted.

## Infant Salmonella

The third story within this case study stemmed from an unusually high incidence of cases of a rare form of *Salmonella* in babies between November 1996 and January 1997. (Twelve cases in the three months, compared with typically one reported case every two or three months.) None of these cases proved fatal, but two involved hospitalization. In January 1997 laboratory tests showed conclusively that ten of the 12 cases involved a distinctive strain of the *Salmonella* 'bug', and that all ten of the babies concerned had been fed with Milupa's 'Milumil' brand of formula.

The government and Milupa responded very quickly. Within 24 hours the product had been withdrawn from sale and press releases had been issued by both the Department of Health (DH) and the manufacturer explaining the situation. The DH cascaded information to medical professionals, and also issued a food hazard warning to environmental health directors, asking them to notify Environmental Health Officers and check that the withdrawal had been put into effect. Milupa established a task force to investigate the incident, and decided completely to relaunch the product after making wide-ranging changes. A month later, after close liaison between Milupa and the DoH, the product was completely relaunched with new formulation, new packaging, a new country of manufacture, and new instructions for preparation.

Thousands of calls were received on the helpline established by Milupa, and by doctors, health visitors, and other professionals. But the advance briefing and prompt, clear action appear to have worked well, and there was no accusation of any cover-up or inadequacy in the government's and Milupa's response. Fergus Walsh, on the BBC 6 O'clock News, commented:

> 'Unlike on previous occasions, this time information was distributed promptly to health professionals to help them deal with enquiries from the public'.

## Dioxins and PCBs

The final story in this case study related to the levels of dioxins and PCBs (polychlorinated biphenyls) in breast milk. These chemicals are widely present at low levels in the environment and in foods, and accumulate in fatty tissues when eaten. High levels fed to laboratory animals have been shown to lead to a wide variety of adverse health effects including increased cancer risk for the animals exposed, reduced fertility, and transmission of impairments to their offspring.

Breast milk is one of the 'foods' of greatest concern in respect of PCBs and dioxins. The chemicals accumulate in fatty tissues (including the breast) through a mother's lifetime exposure to the low levels in foods. On breast feeding, the stored fatty substances are mobilized, releasing some of the PCBs and dioxins (and any other fat-soluble contaminants) into breast milk. The effect is particularly pronounced for first babies; after a period of feeding the concentrations of fat-soluble contaminants in the breast tissue will have decreased.

In April 1997, the government's advisory Committee on Toxicity published a review of PCBs and dioxins in foods which included the information from recent analysis of breast milk samples that some babies could be receiving levels above the tolerable daily intakes, although levels in foods generally were declining. The Department of Health was very sensitive to the potential impact of this news on breast-feeding mothers, and took pains to communicate the risk and its advice, that 'breast was still best'. A press release was issued after briefings to medical professionals and parents' group representatives, and the relevant information and advice was cascaded to health professionals in advance. The media and public response to the issue was very balanced, with apparent general acceptance of the idea that there could be a small risk which was outweighed by the benefit of breast feeding in comparison with other options.

The overall view of officials in DH and MAFF (who now work together in a joint organization in this area) was that they had learnt a lot through these episodes about how to communicate food risk information more effectively to the public. This view was shared by medical, consumer and parents' groups outside government, with the qualification that there was still much progress to be made, and that they would like to be involved in developing the advice, not just in being briefed once policy had been established.

The case study highlighted the importance of involving and informing those to whom the public would turn for advice and guidance in the event of a health scare. It also illustrated the importance of processes and systems in cases where there is a need to get information quickly to a network of professionals who may be deluged with requests for help and advice.

## Land use planning

This case study examined the communication issues surrounding the planning process in connection with hazardous installations—either for developments of hazardous plant, or for property and land use developments within the defined special planning zones around hazardous plant.

The decisions on these issues are made by local planning authorities— elected officials, supported by professional planning teams. Certain planning situations (typically of the order of a thousand each year) must be referred to the Health and Safety Executive (HSE) for advice. The HSE bases its advice on the levels of risk involved in comparison with reference criteria, which are themselves the subject of vigorous consultation and debate with planners and others. But there is no obligation on the local planners to follow this advice; the decision at the end of the day is in the hands of locally accountable representatives.

The HSE is thus in the position, often several times each day, of communicating advice based upon risk assessment to an audience of local decision-makers, who may have little or no special understanding of the technicalities of risk and risk assessment. Some planning authorities are happy to take the HSE advice as definitive, and would seldom, if ever, challenge it against an application. Others, particularly in areas where there is a high density of hazardous installations and a correspondingly high rate of referrals for HSE advice, are much more likely to want to test and challenge the HSE advice and make their own decisions.

The case study examined some of the research carried out into local authority views and how effectively risk advice was communicated to them by the HSE. In the past, there had been many complaints and concerns that the HSE did not understand planning, was unresponsive and slow, and that advice needed to be more definitive ('yes' or 'no', rather than 'maybe if . . .').

While some planners still feel that there is a communication gulf between risk experts from the HSE and local officials ('things would be better if they focused on helping us make difficult decisions, rather than on discussions about criteria'), the general view is that the HSE has improved significantly over the years since these problems were diagnosed. Some of the improvement is down to greater mutual understanding and appreciation of the issues among the HSE inspectors who get involved, some to very simple things such as focusing on the process for logging and acting on requests for advice to ensure quicker turn-around times.

This case study illustrated the scope for relatively simple improvements in the process to make a significant difference to people's satisfaction with the regulatory system, and the value of building up a cadre of people with experience in communicating with the relevant audience. But it also flagged up an important divergence of views about the institutional arrangements whereby regulators support individuals and groups making their own decisions about risk issues which can probably be generalized. Some people want straightforward, simple advice on what to do and what to avoid. Others want to make up their own minds, and expect regulators to provide help in doing so.

These different preferences could lead to two quite different models for 'advisory' regulation. In one model, the regulator advises on what to do and what not to do, using criteria designed to reflect the views, values, and preferences of those affected. In the other model, the regulator makes no such judgements about views and preferences, but facilitates individuals or groups making up their own minds, providing risk information and advice to which people can apply their own criteria.

## Organophosphate use in agriculture

Organophosphate compounds are widely used in agriculture, both as crop pesticides and as veterinary medicines. For a considerable period they were the only approved substances available to be used for sheep dipping, which was mandatory from 1976 to 1992. By their very nature, these compounds are very toxic to people; the health effects following high levels of exposure are well understood, but there has been much controversy over health effects at very low levels of exposure.

The issues associated with pesticide or veterinary medicine use include the health of the public and farmers, and environmental impacts as well as animal and crop welfare. Several different government departments and agencies are thus involved in regulation and enforcement activity. These activities are coordinated through dedicated agencies of MAFF— the Pesticide Safety Directorate (PSD) for crop pesticides, and the Veterinary Medicines Directorate (VMD) for veterinary medicines such as sheep dips.

This case study compared some recent experiences of PSD and VMD in dealing with the impacts of organophosphates on human health. The arrangements for controlling risks are broadly similar in both cases, and include licensing products for sale, advice and guidance on safe use, regulation and enforcement of proper use and disposal, and schemes to deal with suspected adverse human health effects. The case study examined the recent history of development of these arrangements, focusing in particular on the continuing concerns of people who believe they are suffering from health effects due to past exposure to sheep dip, and on the issue of variability of pesticide levels in carrots (and other fruit and vegetables), with the implication that some individual carrots may contain levels above the recommended maximum.

Concerns over sheep dipping, and the possibility of high levels of pesticides in individual carrots, have each led to changes in the arrangements for controlling risks. The case study followed these changes and people's response to them, as judged from media comment. While the two issues are very different, some striking similarities and differences were observed.

The first obvious similarity is the inherent uncertainty involved in linking cause to effect when adverse health effects are suspected of being linked to low levels of exposure to toxic chemicals. Difficulties include estimating the exposure to the chemicals, particularly when this was in the distant past, and getting an accurate diagnosis of the medical condition—it can be very difficult for doctors to distinguish health effects due to toxic substances where the symptoms could have a variety of other causes.

Another similarity noted was the importance of communication in the whole package of measures for controlling the risks—from labelling and advice to farmers, through to strong publicity to promote safe use and disposal (very difficult to enforce on thousands of farms all over the country), to advice to the public about how they can contribute to reducing their own exposure, for example by topping and peeling carrots.

Some of the most striking differences between the two issues examined (other than the inherent difference between exposure to chemicals on farms and by eating food containing residues) were in presentation. While responses to presentation are inevitably subjective, three differences struck the author as being of particular relevance to establishing public confidence and trust.

1. The priority given to public disclosure and information in the Food and Environmental Protection Act of 1985 (governing pesticide use and actively promoting openness) is very different from that in the Medicines Act of 1968 (governing veterinary medicines and, for example, prohibiting

public disclosure of the documents relating to product licensing without specific ministerial approval).

2. The regimes for investigating incidents of suspected ill health have some significant differences. The different nature of the issues means that a high proportion of reported pesticide adverse reactions can be resolved one way or the other to establish whether there was a link between exposure and health effects, whereas for health effects suspected of being due to long-past exposure to sheep dip chemicals it is almost impossible to establish such a causal link. This is absolutely logical and reasonable given the nature of the issues, but the appearance is of regimes which are rather successful in tracking down exposure to people or wild animals due to pesticide use, but hopeless at linking sheep dip to some serious health effects in people.

3. The published information related to these reporting schemes is very differently presented. For veterinary medicines, the investigations of the specialist expert panel are made publicly available in the form of an annual report, simply presented on plain paper and in scientific language. For pesticides, glossy professionally prepared reports are produced with the public audience much more in mind—straightforward explanations of the issues are provided in non-specialist terms, and summary information is digested and attractively presented.

Finally, the sheep dip history in particular demonstrated very clearly how an issue can remain contentious for a very long time when there is an inherent mismatch between the objectives of government scientists working on it, and of those who feel they have been affected by it. The aim of suspected adverse reaction schemes is to establish whether there is a link between exposure and effects, whereas people who feel they have been affected feel that the aim of government schemes should be to help them. Despite all the measures over the years to tighten up on organophosphate use and the depth and sincerity of scientific investigations, there remains a fundamental difference of view between people who think they have suffered from past exposure to sheep dip and the government, as to the link between sheep dip exposure and health.

# Principles for good practice

Based on the literature review and case study observations, the project proposed four principles for governmental good practice in risk communication. They were deliberately kept very simple, and framed so as to cover the entire scope of risk communication in relation to regulation:

- the place of communication in regulation of risks
- the inputs to government in terms of risk communication
- the outputs from government in terms of risk communication
- the process of risk communication within government activity.

## *Principle 1: Integrate risk communication and risk regulation*

Engagement and dialogue with those interested in and affected by risk issues is vital. It should be an integral part of every process for the management and/or regulation of risks. Communication should neither be treated as a bolt-on extra, nor approached solely in the context of one-way provision of public information. The aims of risk communication should be to enable effective participation and/or representation of all interested and affected parties in making decisions about how to manage risks, and to support the most effective possible implementation of risk management decisions.

## *Principle 2: Listen to stakeholders*

Regulatory bodies should identify and engage with all those interested in and affected by each risk issue. They should seek to understand their attitudes to risks and risk control measures. Their views and preferences should be incorporated into policy and practice. Where practicable and appropriate, those affected should be involved in or empowered to take decisions about risks and their control.

## *Principle 3: Tailor the messages*

Government messages and communications about risk should be tailored to their audience and purpose. Particular attention should be paid to:

- engaging and demonstrating empathy with the audience
- displaying openness and responsiveness to audience emotions, fears, and concerns
- demonstrating credibility, competence, and commitment
- articulating the benefits of proposed and/or alternative options for the audience.

## *Principle 4: Manage the process*

Risk communication is always important for policy success. Thus, clear, well-defined risk communication management processes and procedures are needed. These should cover setting goals, allocating responsibilities, planning, implementing, monitoring, and evaluation.

The first and over-arching principle is that communication should be fully integrated with risk regulatory activity. This principle is strategic in nature, with substantial implications for how things are done in government departments and agencies. The other three are more tactical in nature.

# Observations on current practice

The project offered some specific observations on the current status of government practice with respect to each of the four principles.

## Principle 1: Integrate risk communication and risk regulation

With noble exceptions such as the drink-driving programme, government was considered notably weak in this area. Risk communication is generally a 'bolt-on' once the important matters of substance and science have been dealt with. While many people in government at all levels recognize the importance of communication in determining regulatory success, there is little evidence that its importance has been reflected in the way departments go about their regulatory business.

## Principle 2: Listen to stakeholders

In respect of this principle:

- there is fast-growing awareness of its importance and examples of its application;
- practice varies widely across and even within departments, for example on consultation;
- there is generally a 'one way' information flow culture, rather than a focus on two-way dialogue.

Overall, there is significant scope for improvement in government practice here. There is a tide already flowing in this direction which should be recognized and encouraged.

## Principle 3: Tailor the messages

In respect of this principle:

- there are some good developments in progress, e.g. the appointment of consumer representatives onto expert committees, and recent initiatives to integrate health and food safety regulation providing a stronger and more coherent focus for communication; but
- the way government uses expert committees often gives the appearance of passing decisions to scientists rather than bringing together scientific information and social values and preferences; and

- the dominance of science in risk policy tends to lead to objective statements devoid of empathy or emotional content, to a consistent focus on risk reduction rather than on trust and confidence, and to very weak articulation of benefits of proposed risk controls in terms meaningful to audiences.

The overall impression was that this is an area where current government practice is very weak, and where there are major short-term opportunities for improvement.

### Principle 4: Manage the process

The general observation here was that where risk communication has been recognized, legitimized, and resourced, communications management practice in government is good or is improving rapidly. The real issue here is thus the recognition of the importance of the issue (Principle 1); government departments are perfectly capable of managing appropriate risk communications processes and have many opportunities for 'quick wins'.

## Further comments

Overall impressions, based not only on the literature review and case studies but also on numerous interactions with interest groups, commercial organizations, and other researchers and interested parties throughout the project, were as follows.

1.  *Things are getting better* – in all the case studies following progress over a period of time, both government officials and independent parties outside government felt that positive progress had been made over recent years.

2.  Communication is increasingly being used by government as a *risk control policy instrument in its own right*, to influence people towards less risky or better-controlled behaviour in their own interests and that of others.

3.  The government's approach to risk management and regulation is generally *strongly science based*, which has a number of important corollaries:

    – the choice of risk control arrangements is based on ensuring that risks are kept to low, objectively defined levels, established through science with little input of people's views and preferences;

    – the heavy influence of scientists and expert committees provides an inherent barrier to public understanding and engagement; and

-   much of the government's delivery of information about risks is
    framed in a scientific context, on the basis that the importance of
    risk and the choice of arrangements to control risk can be related
    directly to objective measures of likelihood and of consequences.
    Most people do not share this reference framework. To many
    people, the government's approach thus comes across as dry and
    unemotive, focused on science and not on people.

4.  Communication *still tends to be a 'bolt on'* to mainstream risk regulation
    and policy issues, rather than being an integral part.

5.  Communication has been institutionalized in much of government as
    'information'. Thus every department has an information unit, and
    employs communications professionals typically under a 'Head of
    Information'. Their role is well understood, and procedures are in place
    to ensure their very considerable expertise is utilized whenever infor-
    mation is being issued from the department. Provision of information is
    clearly an important issue and duty for government. *But the focus on
    information, rather than communication, implies a one-way approach.* A
    change of culture, from 'information provision' to 'two-way commu-
    nication' is a principal theme of the study's recommendations.

In summary, there is much good practice in risk communication in
government on which to draw, and evidence of positive progress in recent
years. There are also some important weaknesses, substantial opportunities,
and a strong appetite for improvement.

---

## REFERENCES

Department of the Environment (1976). Drinking and Driving. Report of the
    Departmental Committee on Drinking and Driving (chairman F. Blennerhassett).
    HMSO, London.
Health and Safety Executive (1998). *Risk communication—benchmarking in govern-
    ment*. Health and Safety Executive, London.

# PART 3

## Institutional issues: some perspectives

### Preface to Part 3

The next six chapters bring together a range of perspectives on political and institutional dimensions of risk communication. They juxtapose contributions from a senior government scientist, the former chair of a prominent scientific advisory committee, and campaigners for environmental and consumer concerns. These are followed by some specific proposals for improving 'openness' and participation in the policy process, and some actions already in train.

We start with a contribution from David Fisk, Chief Scientist at the Department of the Environment, Transport and the Regions. His thesis—which might once have been regarded as somewhat heretical from such a source—is that the public is more often right about risks than regulators are prone to suppose. Interestingly, this conclusion is reached not by invoking more fashionable arguments from social science but by applying traditional risk assessment *from a citizen's perspective*. Seeing public concerns as defensible provides one argument for opening up the regulatory process to wider participation. This is a theme running strongly through all the following chapters.

As the British scientific advisory committee system features extensively in the following discussion, a brief introduction may be helpful. The committees are an important feature of the regulatory system. They are composed of independent experts—with a predominance of prestigious academics—rather than civil servants or government employees. Nevertheless, they are established by ministers or (in the health field) the Chief Medical Officer and supported by a secretariat within the appropriate department. There are standing committees covering major policy areas (for example the regulation of novel foods, the medical effects of air pollution, or the safety of medicines), while others are set up to deal with particular one-off issues. In either case, the aim is to obtain independent, authoritative advice, particularly where the science itself may be unclear or contentious. (More 'routine' cases are more usually analysed by a department's own scientific staff.) A committee's report should represent a consensus view of experts of national—and frequently international—standing, and take account of the full range of relevant scientific data and opinion. Individual committees have broader or narrower remits. Some focus on scientific issues, for example in examining the evidence base to identify the nature of a hazard, the extent of public exposure, and its possible medical effects given current knowledge. Others may also be expected to consider the wider implications of a potential hazard, taking account of ethical issues and other public concerns. Sometimes ministers have asked for direct advice on policies for managing a hazard—for example, the Spongiform Encephalopathy Advisory Committee (SEAC) on specific occasions in relation to BSE/CJD.

In Chapter 11, Derek Burke describes how one key committee has sought to engage a wide variety of viewpoints in dealing with the issue of genetically modified food. Ian Taylor of Greenpeace UK uses a case study in the same area to argue the need for further reform of the regulatory system, particularly at a European level, in order to foster a more precautionary approach. Sheila McKechnie and Sue Davies of the Consumers' Association stress the need for consumer involvement in matters such as food safety. Chiming in with earlier contributions, all reiterate the loss of public confidence in traditional mechanisms of both government and science, and the need to respond with new participative measures. Anna Coote and Jane Franklin recapitulate the problems and suggest the use of Citizens' Juries as one participative mechanism, drawing on work carried out by the Institute for Public Policy Research. Finally in Chapter 15, David Coles of the Department of Health discusses current developments in opening up the British regulatory system, bringing a continuing story up to date (as of August 1998), and reflects on experiences in other countries.

# 10 Perception of risk—is the public probably right?

David Fisk
*Chief Scientist, DETR[1]*

## Introduction

The Royal Society's seminal review of risk management (Royal Society 1992) brought together three views of the problem of risk. The first might be termed the *pure engineering* view: risk is a quantity to be calculated from hard data. The second might be termed the *psychometric* or *economist's* view: subjects filter the engineering risks of the 'real world' into perceived problems. The third view is typically that of the *anthropologist* or *sociologist*: risk is a problem in a wider context of relationships within society. The last two in particular are explored by other contributors to this volume.

For those trying to improve public decision-making in environmental policy, the key question is whether these different perspectives lead to different *recommendations*. I will argue that in fact they lead to similar recommendations for the preferred participative process. Specifically, I will pick the most traditional approach, that of the engineer, and show that this risk methodology actually predicts a plurality of risk assessments by different rational participants. Furthermore, it predicts how to design processes which improve the chances of the perspectives converging. Perhaps surprisingly, the recommendations would look very familiar to adherents of the social science approach. Properly applied, an engineering point of view suggests that in many cases 'the public is probably right'. In other words, a traditional form of analysis leads towards some rather radical-sounding conclusions.

1. The views expressed are those of the author and do not necessarily represent those of the Department of the Environment, Transport and the Regions.

# Cognitive versus sensory perception

At the outset, we need to be clear how a plurality of views arises. Although we frequently talk of the perception of risk, there is more than one meaning of 'perception'. *Sensory* perception applies to responses to stimuli like noise or light. Similarly we can perceive small numbers of objects—like two or three—without resorting to counting. But for larger figures our perception is more likely to be *cognitive*. We perceive large numbers by thinking of a process ('if all the risk analysts in the world were laid end to end ...'). Similarly for small probabilities of 'one in a large number'. Some risk situations may have high probabilities, and so may be argued to fall under sensory perception (like the 50:50 chance of a tossed coin coming up heads). But in environmental policy, the probabilities of adverse events tend, fortunately, to be very small. They are typically one event in $10^4$ per annum or rarer. These are a very long way from familiar betting odds. It therefore seems reasonable to assume that understanding of such low risks is largely cognitive. Small probabilities are *conceived*, not directly *perceived*. It is therefore not surprising that participants who bring different mental processes to bear—notably regulators and the regulated—will come to have very different understandings of risks. An understanding of how reasoning might have diverged is a first step towards identifying how convergence towards a social consensus could be encouraged. The following sections look at two sources of divergence.

# Different sampling

A simple form of divergence between regulated and regulator can arise because each is legitimately sampling from a different world. Citizens may not wish to fault the regulators' logic, but observe that the assumptions used do not apply to their particular case. Thus the statutory duty of a regulator might be cast in terms of protecting society on average, not a member of the public in particular. While citizens may have a passing interest in risks faced by others, their principal concern is likely to be personal risk (to themselves, close family, etc.). A passage in the Royal Society report (1992) provides a good example of how these perspectives may diverge in the context of transport risks.

Chapter 4 of the report offers a discussion of the use of comparative risk tables. The example chosen is the risk of a fatality travelling from one location in the UK to another. From the transport regulator point of view, fatalities per passenger kilometre are lower for air (on scheduled airlines) than any other mode of transport. This might suggest that this is the safest way to travel. But is this the most appropriate measure for the individual traveller to use? Air accidents are dominated by problems on taking off and landing. It follows that a longer trip averages lower accidents per kilometre than a short trip, an effect not present for car or train. Individual travellers will know into which class their journey falls. Meanwhile the comparative riskiness of road travel is influenced by whether the car or bus driver is under the influence of alcohol. The official statistics cited in the Royal Society report average out these differences. However, it is easy for the individual citizen to determine whether the journey would fall into the higher-risk, drunken driver category (try saying 'good morning' to the driver: the case is even more self-evident if you are driving yourself!). Local information may therefore lead to decisions that are perfectly rational, yet inconsistent with a regulator's averaged view—even if risk minimization is the sole concern of both sides.

# Expert error

Even if the regulator/expert has been invited to address the risk issue from an individual citizen's point of view, the rational citizen might still wish to introduce some risk discount. This arises because expert processes are as prone to error as any other. A rational citizen can quite legitimately apply a further discount in the same way that a regulator would apply a discount for 'operator error' when assessing processing plant safety. We consider three reasons for such discounts.

## Experts underestimate risk of error

While regulators are well armed with the probability of *other people* making errors, they are notably thin on estimating the probability that they themselves are in error. Revisiting early estimates of important physical constants is informative. While, as to be expected, early estimates are usually given with much wider 'standard errors' than those found by later, more refined techniques, there is a consistent bias to underestimate the errors. Errors in 'confident' medical opinion, gathered from when a disease was first characterized, are typically so wide that no-one appears to have had the heart to catalogue them. An individual is therefore perfectly entitled to impose a risk discount to expert advice to allow for possible over-confidence.

## Experts do not bear risks

It would be normal engineering risk assessment practice to expect the risk of error to vary with the incentive to be right. The citizen would be quite rational to adjust a regulator's risk assessment depending on whether the regulator bore any personal accountability if the hazard were realized. Assessing the credibility of expert judgement of risk is not a new problem. For thousands of years the approach has been to address the problem through the management of *risk transfer*. When building construction was at the cutting edge of new technology, societies had to handle the risks of new structures such as the arch. In Babylon any fatalities to slaves or family from a building collapse entitled the building owner to exact a similar penalty from the architect's household. In Roman practice both the architect and building contractor stood together underneath an arch when the formwork was removed. In contrast, modern advisory committees usually ask for professional indemnity before they offer an opinion!

Now, Parliament may give governments the power to remedy errors of regulatory function, but they seldom make it a duty. Legal codes may even bias the burden of proof in a regulatory decision, for example in favour of 'economic development'. There is nothing wrong in principle with any of these decisions—as long as they are not taken covertly. After all, a committee of volunteers prepared to be decapitated if its judgement is wrong would not necessarily be the best mentally-balanced for assisting the regulatory process. Nevertheless, a citizen is quite right to apply a risk discount to the regulatory position to allow for the different views of burden of proof.

## Precompression of risk

Regulators and advisory committees do indeed make real world errors. One type is so prevalent that it deserves special mention. This is to confuse 'no evidence' with 'evidence not'. When an advisory committee cannot find any evidence of harm, this may be because the concern is groundless, but it may be because the detection techniques are not sufficiently powerful to detect the effects. Experts are always under severe pressure to compress discordant facts into simple outcomes. Clients are unlikely to fund an expert a second time if the answer they got the first time was that the client's guess was as good as any! If experts reject the existence of effects when current methods are insensitive, or otherwise filter data before a risk analysis stage, they will be led to a flawed final conclusion. Only a few countries have in place the mechanisms to ensure that these errors are spotted in expert processes. Such guidance does exist in the UK (the so-called *May Guidance*), but dates only from 1997.

# Risk management and the citizen

The foregoing analysis leads to a number of conclusions on how to minimize unnecessary divergence in citizen and expert views of risk. However, much of the inherent idea that 'the public is probably wrong' does not stem from citizens' *declared* personal risk analysis. Rather, it stems from regulators observing what citizens actually do. As a coda, I will therefore explore why rational citizen behaviour will sometimes appear irrational to the regulator. There are a number of reasons why this should be so. The behaviour of the individual may reflect more than the presence of risk. It may reflect the politics of risk being transferred from one party to another, with or without compensation. It may reflect a rational inclination to avoid a risk—no matter how small—if avoidance carries no cost. It may also reflect other values that are altered by the presence of risk. I will illustrate each point briefly.

## Risk management is a political process

In environmental policy, risk management is essentially a political process. It involves moving risks from one party and imposing them on another. In these circumstances it is not too surprising that individuals may object on 'fairness' grounds to the newly imposed risk. This is not strictly a *risk* perception.

## Risk management at the margin

Though decisions by individual citizens may have profound effects on those who supply them with goods and services, the decision itself (say choosing between different bottled mineral waters) may be of trivial significance to the citizen. So it would be rational to avoid an option differing from the others only in a minute risk of (say) one in $10^{30}$. To any regulator brought up on the notion that a one in $10^6$ risk was 'tolerable', this could look highly irrational.

## Risk exposure as a 'good'

A risk is an attribute not only of the hazard concerned, but of associated economic goods. A foodstuff that is in the news with health scares has a different 'quality' from one marketed as being from 'traditional' sources—especially when being chosen as the main course for a dinner party. A house next to a waste tip has more to contend with in the housing market than just the low risk of contamination. Elements of choice that relate to 'positional' goods may easily be confused with assessments of risk.

# Opening up risk assessment

The preceding arguments show that even classical engineering risk analysis predicts a plurality of views about the risks presented by a hazard, and a plurality of 'rational' responses. However, they also suggest a few easy steps to minimize the differences. At a number of stages in the analysis, I suggested that it is rational for the citizen to apply additional risk factors to cover areas of uncertainty. However, much of that uncertainty is (from the citizen's point of view) an unnecessary product of the regulatory process, particularly its lack of openness.

## Open access to raw data

My first suggestion was that individual citizens might use that same data as the regulator but draw different conclusions in different circumstances. If regulators only present their data in particular normalizations (e.g. fatalities per passenger kilometre) this provokes a social division between regulator and citizens. If the latter have access to the underlying data (e.g. number of accidents, number of accidents per fatality, etc.) at least the debate will have the appearance of starting from a common base. The absence of raw data from which to calculate individual viewpoints provokes the citizen to exaggerate the difference between his/her own judgements and that given by the regulator's calculation.

## Open processes

My second conclusion was that the citizen, using traditional risk analysis, could legitimately apply a risk factor to cover error by the regulator. Regulators should be as keen as everyone else to reduce the need for this factor as much as possible. They will normally have tough *internal* audit processes. But opening these procedures to the public provides further re-assurance that errors or omissions have not been made. Public access, of course, need not be the same as publication. Some reassurance may be gained by knowing that an assessment was drawn up in the full knowledge that it might be made public.

## Strict process guidance

Logical errors in handling scientific data are common in risk analysis. To encourage citizens to reduce their estimate of the likelihood of error, regulatory bodes and their advisory machinery need to work to clear process guidance. As far as possible it should separate assessing the science (what we know and what we do not know) from risk analysis.

## Clear statement of scope of risk assessment

Where risk assessments imply transfers of risk between citizens, the transfers need to be explicit. This involves making clear which risks are included in the assessment to be offset against each other, and where a burden of proof is being assigned in one direction or another.

# Final comments

The conclusions set out here align with other approaches concerned to advance the participative process. They emphasize that in its own terms 'the public is probably right'. The steps suggested will improve the social consensus, but they do not guarantee harmony. The regulator may perform the role of informing the citizen, or may facilitate a bargain between different citizens where risk is being transferred. But the regulator may also be required to strike a balance between parties with different interests. Taking into account what traditional risk theory has to say about minimizing differences helps, but it does not remove the underlying politics.

## REFERENCES

The Royal Society (1992). *Risk analysis, perception and management*. The Royal Society, London.

May, R. (1997). The Use of Scientific Advice in Policy Making. Department of Trade and Industry, London.

# 11 The recent excitement over genetically modified foods

Derek Burke
*Chairman, Advisory Committee on Novel Foods and Processes*
*1988–1997*

## What is the problem?

Over the last two years, genetically modified foods have been entering
supermarkets in Britain as a result of the regulatory decisions made by
the committee which I chaired for nine years, the Advisory Committee on
Novel Foods and Processes (ACNFP). The outcome has been mixed; some
products have been accepted without hesitation by the public, 'vegetarian
cheese' and the paste made from genetically modified tomatoes come to
mind, but others, notably the flour from genetically modified soya beans
and an insect-resistant corn have caused considerable controversy, and
the consequences have reached right up to the top of decision-making in
the EU and in some of its member states. Why is this, and what is the cause
of the public's concern? I will try to explain what I think is happening,
using some of the modified foods that have come to ACNFP for approval
as examples, but first I will describe the structure and function of the
committee.

## The current regulatory process

The ACNFP is an independent advisory committee, made up of 16 experts
in different areas—genetic manipulation, microbiology, toxicology, nutrition, plant breeding, etc. It also has a consumer representative and an ethical
advisor. To date, it has approved just over 50 products, 16 of which have
been products of genetic modification, although not all of them are on the
market. It might be useful to briefly summarize them, as follows:

*Foods obtained through genetic modification*

    Enzymes, such as chymosin, from three different sources.

    Oils from genetically modified crops such as rape, maize, and soya.

    Herbicide-resistant crops such as soya and rape.

    Tomatoes and tomato paste.

*Non-genetically modified novel foods*

    Mycoprotein.

    Speciality oils.

    Modified fats and sugars.

    Novel cereals such as lupin.

    Microorganisms such as *Lactobacillus*.

Most of the public's attention has concentrated on the foods obtained through genetic modification, and it is in this area that we have had most to learn.

The committee worked initially on a case-by-case basis, but later systematized this process into a series of decision trees, consulting widely as it developed the process. It used the concept of *substantial equivalence*, which involves a detailed comparison with the non-modified food. The committee looks not only for any direct changes, but also for any *indirect* changes, caused for example by any perturbing effect on metabolism. It invariably needed to go back to the company for further information, including raw data if appropriate, and further experimental work was often needed. Thus, the committee conducts a full scientific risk evaluation. Once satisfied, the committee *recommends to* ministers, who have always accepted the advice, and who then issue government approval.

We used to think, we experts, that all we had to do was to decide whether a novel food or process was safe or not and a grateful public would accept what we said. We should have known better! Food irradiation, a process I, and many others, believe to be safe, is unusable because of fears connected with the word 'irradiation', going back to the atomic bomb and fed by concerns about nuclear power stations. That should have made us think again. When the committee started, it had not grasped the very different way the consumer sees risk.

# Learning the hard way

We learned our first lesson in late 1988, when asked to approve the use of a genetically modified baker's yeast developed by introducing two genes from a similar yeast in order to increase the rate at which the bread rose. This seemed a good case with which to start. After all, the genetic change could have been brought about by the naturally occurring yeast mating process. The committee could not see any problem, and in early 1990, a brief press release appeared which announced that 'the product may be used safely'. The press reactions were not enthusiastic, and varied from 'Genetic yeast passed for use' in *The Times*, through 'Man-made yeast raises temperature' in *The Independent*, to 'Bionic bread sales wrapped in secrecy' in *Today*, and 'Are the boffins taking the rise out of bread?' in *The Star*! The Consumers' Association said: 'We think all genetically altered foods should be labelled' and the general reaction was so negative that the product has never been used.

The committee dealt with this setback by gathering together, for a weekend conference, representatives of all the groups who might be able to help avoid this problem in future. This included scientists, social scientists (especially to help over risk assessment), civil servants, a philosopher, a churchman, and representatives from several alternative groups. As a result, a number of recommendations were made to ministers, which were accepted, and the procedure changed substantially. So, six years ago, a consumer representative and an ethical advisor were added to the committee. I believe that this was the first time that such representatives were members of a specialist Government Advisory Committee, although this practice has now become widespread. We also took a number of steps to open up the process and make it more transparent. For some years now the committee has produced an annual report and held an annual press conference. Press releases are produced before and after each meeting of the ACNFP, as well as after ministerial approval of each product or process. The chairman sees, and sometimes rewords, the press releases—and also make a point of being available to reporters for newspapers, radio, and television. All these changes have been in place for some years now, and have been the basis of all our subsequent decisions. We have learned that when decisions involve the public being exposed to any risk not of its own choosing, they must be taken as openly as possible.

About five years ago the committee was asked whether meat from genetically modified sheep could enter the food chain. These sheep carried the human gene for Factor IX, a protein needed for the treatment of haemophiliacs. However, it often takes 100 animals to be reared before one animal is produced which yields Factor IX in high quantities. The committee was asked about the animals which either contained no gene, or only an inactive gene or part of a gene. Could they be eaten? It could not think of any reason why animals without any foreign DNA should not be eaten. But were newspapers going to run the headline: 'Failures from genetic engineering in your supermarket'?. What about the animals containing an inactive human gene? Was this just a stretch of DNA like any other? Or was it special because it came from a human being? Would eating sheep meat containing a single human gene even be regarded as cannibalism by some? Would Muslims or Jews be concerned about pork genes in lamb, and vegetarians about animal genes in plants? The committee did not know, but decided that it was probably a wider issue than one of pure technical safety, and suggested to the minister that there should be wider consultation. The minister agreed and a small committee was set up under the chairmanship of the Reverend John Polkinghorne KBE, FRS. I was also a member of that committee.

This committee found that the Christians were divided. Some had no objections, but many had an uneasy concern, a feeling shared by others, which has been termed the 'yuk' factor. The Jewish reaction was more straightforward: 'If it looks like a sheep, then it is a sheep' was their comment. Muslims and Hindus were much more opposed, as were the animal welfare groups and the vegetarians. None of the groups were moved when it was pointed out that there was effectively no chance of their eating the original human gene, for it was hugely diluted in the processes of genetic manipulation, and the gene inserted into the sheep was more correctly called a 'copy gene'. They were even concerned if the gene was completely synthetic. They were also concerned by the 'slippery slope' argument. These sheep had only one human gene in 100 000 sheep genes. But what if it was 50:50? Then it is likely that all of us would be concerned. They were worried too about labelling, and wanted consumers to have choice. There was obviously quite widespread unease. The committee made a series of recommendations, which were accepted, with the result that not even the animals without any foreign genes will enter the food chain. Consumer concerns, even if they do not appear to have a rational basis to scientists, must be taken seriously and not brushed away.

The committee has found that scientific and consumer issues are best settled side-by-side, not consecutively as they used to be. The previous approach: 'First sort out the science and then look at the consumer issues' simply does not work in our experience. A lesson learnt first over the baker's yeast, and then over the transgenic sheep, was that the question was not going to be resolved by a purely scientific discussion. In that case a series of scientific questions was asked—about chromosome fragmentation, mosaicism, and the lower limits of detection of gene fragments—that would not have asked but for consumer concerns.

## Plant genetic modification

In plants, the first genes to be manipulated were the herbicide-resistant genes. This is often put down to a 'plot' by the companies concerned to increase their sales of herbicides, and companies were of course aware of that opportunity, for it enabled them to integrate the two formerly separate areas of seed production and pesticide use. However, an equally important reason was that the genes for herbicide resistance are single genes and therefore much easier to isolate and manipulate than the multigene complexes responsible for such important traits as salt tolerance and drought resistance. A number of such herbicide-resistant crops are now being grown.

A number of products from several herbicide-resistant plants have been approved by the committee. Many of these have been quite straightforward, but difficulty has arisen over a line of soya beans from Monsanto that were resistant to the herbicide glyphosate. Glyphosate works by inactivating an enzyme in the plant which is essential for the production of complex amino acids, thereby preventing growth. Glyphosate tolerance was achieved through the introduction of a gene from an *Agrobacterium* into a commercial soya bean cultivar. This gene codes for an enzyme that has the same function as the glyphosate-sensitive enzyme in the plant but is not itself inhibited by glyphosate. The bacterial form of the enzyme therefore remains active in the presence of glyphosate when the plant enzyme is inhibited. The modified soya also contains part of a gene from *Petunia hybrida* which encodes a chloroplast transit peptide responsible for delivering the bacterial enzyme gene to the chloroplasts, the site of aromatic amino acid synthesis in plants. When the enzyme reaches the chloroplast, the attached transit peptide is cleaved and degraded. The committee had no safety concerns over the product, which is the flour rather than the beans, since the DNA is degraded during the production of the flour, and the bacterial enzyme, which is present at very low levels in the soya beans ($< 0.1\%$), did not present any food safety hazard.

## Labelling issues

The Food Advisory Committee decided that the product did not need to be labelled, although information was provided on a voluntary basis by the retailer, as had been done in the successful launch of the paste from genetically modified tomatoes earlier in the year. However, with soya meal, the retailers have not been able to offer customers choice between a modified and an unmodified product, because of the lack of segregation in the United States of the soya crop. This has meant that choice is effectively no longer available to the consumer in the UK, and soya is included as an ingredient in the majority of processed foods. It is not surprising that North American farmers are unwilling to segregate their genetically modified (GM) crops, since there seems to be little demand for segregation in North America, while the costs of segregation would be considerable and would counter any benefit of growing them. The US government has supported the farmers in this stance by clearly stating that any attempt to ban the import of soya or maize would be considered a breach of World Trading Organisation agreements.

So despite the best efforts of the retailers, there has been substantial consumer concern because of the absence of choice. There have been several different types of response; for example, the National Farmers Union has recently launched two complementary codes of practice for the growing of GM crops in the UK which should ultimately allow foods that contain material derived from GM crops to be labelled to ensure consumer choice. In the absence of segregation, a number of companies are developing tests to detect transgenic material so that foods containing modified soya can be labelled. Recently (18 March 1998), the Iceland Group, the frozen food retailer, announced that from 1 May none of its own label products will contain any genetically modified ingredients. This promise depends upon the Group being able to access sufficient non-genetically modified soya for all its own-label products, and this might become difficult if all the major producers switch over to growing genetically modified soya. MAFF has also recently published the names of 48 growers and suppliers of organically modified soya beans in order to help smaller UK food producers to find alternatives to genetically modified soya, and so provide consumer choice. It will be interesting to see how strongly consumers feel about this issue, and specifically whether Iceland's market share increases, for experience with the modified tomato paste in the UK shows that consumers will buy a clearly labelled product of genetic modification, especially when they have choice.

However, the situation over labelling is still unsatisfactory. No doubt stirred by the public dissatisfaction earlier this summer, the European Commissioners proposed a labelling framework for products from GM crops. There were to be three categories. The first, which is *voluntary* labelling, was negative, e.g. 'This does *not* contain material of Genetically Modified Organism (GMO) origin', while the other two were *mandatory* and were either 'This *contains* material of GMO origin', or 'This *may* contain material of GMO origin'. On 31 July 1997 the EU agreed that the rules should also apply to GM products that had already been approved for use in the EU, such as soya and maize. The exact labelling requirements for such products were to have been outlined by the EC in early November, but this has not yet happened. Mainly because of this confusion and delay, the Institute of Grocery Distributors (IGD) announced, on 20 November 1997, that its members were to introduce voluntary labelling guidelines for 1998 for products containing soya. It has decided that products containing soya should be labelled as *'containing'* GM soya. The 'may contain' label is not to be used.

So, given these problems, why is the cultivation of genetically modified crops growing so quickly? Herbicide-resistant soya has real advantages for the farmer. In the US, where spring sowing is normal, the use of a post-emergent herbicide means some changes in agronomic practice, leading to retention of more moisture in the soil. Partly because of this, partly because of the slightly longer growing season, and partly because of the effectiveness of the herbicide Roundup, the yields are significantly higher. I believe these crops are here to stay. For instance, US farmers planted some 1.5 million acres of GM soya beans in 1996, and this rose to about 10 million acres (some 15% of the total US acreage) in 1997, and was predicted to rise to about 40 million acres in 1998. The introduction of these new crops will mean changes in the way farmers work. Monsanto is asking for, and obtaining, an increased price for the genetically modified seed, and also an agreement making it impossible to sell or sow seed from the harvest. The company will also supply the farmer with a card that enables him or her to buy Roundup at a reduced price for use on the crop.

It is extremely unfortunate that Monsanto has taken such an aggressive approach, largely ignoring European consumer concerns. In my view, the way in which this product has been introduced has set back the whole commercial development of plant genetic manipulation in Europe. Consumers do not see why they should lose their ability to choose whether or not to consume a product about which they may have concerns, simply to put money into the pockets of the farmers and the company.

## Antibiotic resistance genes

More recently, there has been concern about antibiotic resistance genes in transformed plants. Were such genes at all likely to be transferred to gut bacteria, and if so, did it matter? The committee recommended approval of a modified tomato, despite it containing an antibiotic resistance gene, because the gene was controlled by a plant promoter, and therefore could not work in gut bacteria, and because the antibiotic, kanamycin, was not of great clinical significance. In contrast, a Ciba-Geigy maize contained, in addition to a bacterial gene (the Bt gene) that confers resistance to the European corn borer and a gene that confers resistance to the herbicide glufosinate-ammonium, a third gene that confers resistance to the antibiotic ampicillin. This third gene has been the source of the trouble, for it has a bacterial promoter in front of the penicillinase gene, and in addition, a high copy number plasmid had been used, while the gene in question produced a particularly active penicillinase. The antibiotic resistance gene was a residue left over from the construction of the original plasmid used for the plant transformation and served no useful function in the plant, because it is inactive in plant cells.

The committee was concerned whether there was any risk of transfer of this antibiotic resistance gene into gut bacteria when the maize was used for animal feed *in an unprocessed form* (processing for animal feed degrades the genes, as shown by PCR analysis, and this type of corn is *not* used for human foodstuffs). The technical risk was certainly small, but the consequential risk could have been large. The committee did not recommend approval of this product, but this decision was later overruled by the EU on a majority vote, the EU food committees considering that the possibility of such a transfer adding significantly to antibiotic resistance in animals and man was remote. They did not consider, therefore, that the risk constituted a sufficient reason for a ban. However, a number of EU members would not accept this decision, because of consumer pressure, and the situation has not yet been resolved. The maize is only to be used as an animal feed, and as a source of starch for food ingredients, and has yet to be imported or grown in Europe, though France was given clearance for Bt maize to be grown in 1998.

The consequences of these problems in food safety have been widespread. Mainly as a result of BSE, but also partly as a result of this difficulty, the supervision of the Brussels food committees have been transferred to DG 24, Consumer Affairs. The British Government is also actively planning the formation of a Food Standards Agency, largely because of the loss of public confidence in the food approval process.

## Consumer values

Why is this? Why do consumers want to make their own decisions? Basically I think because they have lost a lot of confidence in what they hear from politicians and, to a lesser extent, from regulators. And what are the reasons for this loss of consumer confidence? Let me suggest several.

1. Scientists and the expert approval processes are no longer trusted as they once were. The 'man in the white laboratory coat' no longer recommends washing powder; the consumer does. Some of this may be due to a general 'decline of deference', but there other reasons: scientists have sometimes been too influenced by commercial or political pressures, or just by the current of the times.

2. I think the public is largely unaware of the development of careful scientific methods of assessing risk, such as the use of hazard analysis, to

come much closer to an 'objective' evaluation of risk. But it is also true that we find great difficulty in explaining, and the public in understanding, what is meant by different degrees of risk. Our National Lottery with its slogan 'It could be you' does not help either—the message is clear: even what is very unlikely may happen. It has been pointed out that you are more likely to die while watching the National Lottery than win the jackpot, but that doesn't stop people buying tickets; someone has to win! So even if the risk from a new product is very low, maybe it will be me!

3.   The public finds it difficult to know how seriously to take the points put by the many single-issue pressure groups.

4.   Risks are assessed differently according to the context. We will accept quite high risks when we are seriously ill, but will not tolerate much risk at all with food. Medicine is restoring natural function to an organism already threatened, but food is the 'staff of life', a basic good that must not be threatened.

One explanation for such conflicting views is that scientists and the public work from different value systems. Scientists and technologists see novel applications of new discoveries as logical and reasonable, and characterize all opposition as unreasonable. 'If only they understood what we are doing' they say 'the public would agree with us'. Scientists are used to an uncertain world, where knowledge is always flawed, can handle risk judgements more easily, and are impatient of those who differ from them. The public's reaction is quite different, and it can be described as:

*Outrage*: 'how dare they do this to us?';

*Dread*: the way we would regard a nuclear power station explosion;

*Stigma*: the way the public regard food irradiation.

So scientists are regarded as arrogant, distant, and uncaring. That's not a good image for science or for scientists.

There is another concern expressed by the public: some think that scientists are playing God. The public asks 'how do you know you are not going to release a new plague?' Scientists reply that they see living systems as a unity, knowing that cells from bacteria to man work in much the same way. So of course it's all right to move genes around—all we have to do is to explain it clearly and people will be reassured. We are not abusing our position as the most powerful species. We know what we are doing.

I think this is all too glib. There are, first of all, important technical issues to be talked about, particularly environmental issues. Will herbicide resistance spread to weeds; will antibiotic resistance genes transfer from plants to man through gut bacteria? The environmental issues are being carefully regulated by a parallel committee to the one that I chaired, The Advisory Committee on Release into the Environment (ACRE). It is being careful and cautious, insisting on a series of controlled trials— first in a contained greenhouse, then in a carefully isolated field plot—before finally going out to planting. The pollen dispersal and the adjacent flora are being monitored to see if there is any spread of the GM crop. So far it has been all right, but the situation wants careful watching, and concerns have been expressed that the 'case-by-case' approach used by the committee will not deal with the sum of a series of decisions about release. Recently, the Nuffield Council on Bioethics has announced that it is undertaking an enquiry into the ethical concerns expressed about the genetic modification of plants and how those concerns might be met.

There are other issues. There is the natural/unnatural issue. Some think that it is unwise, even unethical, to disturb the natural world—and that genetic modification is unnatural because it crosses species barriers. Others believe that BSE resulted from the 'unnatural' feeding of an animal foodstuff to a herbivore; in their view BSE is a sort of Divine Judgement for upsetting the natural order of things. Personally, I do not accept that all that is natural is best; fungal infection of crops with production of the ergot alkaloids is certainly not for the good of those who eat the crops. And why the yoghurt that I eat for my lunch is better for containing 'natural' colouring defeats me! I personally do not think there is an issue here, but many people do.

But to go back to a fundamental question: why were the people we consulted so resistant to the idea of eating a human gene—even when it was totally synthetic? Partly, I think, because they do not know where to draw the line between one gene and a thousand. Is this the start of a slippery slope? Surely we must be able to draw a line somewhere: I believe that we certainly have to try. We already do so in other cases, for example in the case of experiments on very early human embryos.

But I think there is another reason as well. I suspect that people think there is something special about human genes. Is there a concern about what science is doing to our perception of humanness? People are loving, caring, choosing human beings, with deeply held beliefs and values, many of which are central to their view of what a human being is. They accept the centrality of our genes—but not that we are *no more than* a bunch of genes. So they think that there must be something special about human genes, which must not be treated merely as chemicals. Is this a reaction to reductionism—a rejection of the idea that we are nothing but a bunch of genes? The concern of the public is not lessened by the aggressive determinism of some current biologists or by the slant of some of the science-education initiatives. Calling man 'the third chimpanzee' does not help.

# Lessons to learn

What lessons can we draw from this to guide us for the future? First let me suggest four criteria for the developments of a new product:

- it must be technically possible—and now almost anything is possible
- it must offer the consumer, and not just the producer, an advantage
- the regulatory process must be rigorous, open, and universal
- the consumer must be offered choice, at least for some time.

Given these guidelines, I believe that biotechnology will dominate advances in the food and agricultural industries, provided that the consumer understands and accepts the need for and the safety of the new products and processes.

Then let me sum up the lessons we have learnt about relations with consumers:

- nothing is gained by even appearing to withhold information from the consumer
- when decisions involve the public being exposed to any risk not of their own choosing, they must be taken as openly as possible
- consumer concerns, even if they do not appear to have a rational basis to scientists, must be taken seriously and not brushed aside
- consumers want to make their own, informed decisions.

I believe that as regulators we have three stakeholders: industry, government, and the consumer, and we must meet the reasonable needs of all three if we are to retain their trust. We must work efficiently and effectively with industry, advise governments wisely, and be as open as we can with the consumer. That means, I believe, using a case-by-case approach involving representatives of all the parties. This has been the approach of the 'consensus conferences' that have considered issues in both plant and food biotechnology. This has also been the approach used in the ACNFP.

So how should the ethical issues be handled? These remain, in my view, our biggest unsolved problem. A recent Eurobarometer survey (Wagner et al. 1997) showed that risk issues were generally neutral in the public's attitude to biotechnology 'which centres on questions of moral acceptability', although food production was one of the few cases where risk perception was an issue. Indeed, in my view, the resistance to GM foods by Greenpeace and the animal welfare groups springs from ethical concerns rather than risk issues. So we will never meet their concerns by just dealing with risk. The approach in the ACNFP has been to have an ethical advisor as a member of the committee, who advises as to whether there is an ethical issue or not, and if there is, then to advise the minister to consult more widely. But whom does the minister consult? My experience is that scientists are rarely of any use for they do not understand consumer concerns. Nor are professional philosophers very helpful, for in Britain most of them seem much more concerned with analysis. I have found it useful to consult social scientists to help me understand consumer concerns, but they can offer less help with their resolution. I have had most help from two sources: theologians, whether from the Anglican, Roman Catholic, or Jewish communities, and the medical profession. These are the people who continue to be involved in the issues that new technology throws up, and we need to talk to them more.

So, in summary, my judgement is that we have now evolved a satisfactory procedure for monitoring the safety of novel foods, but we are still learning how to handle the ethical issues that cause consumers' concern. Behind these two issues lies that of choice. To take soya as an example, I believe that herbicide-resistant soya is perfectly safe, and that many people would not consider there to be an ethical issue here. But consumers may still, for other reasons, decide that they do not want to eat such soya. If possible, they should have choice, but if that is impracticable, then we should label.

---

## REFERENCE

---

Wagner, W. *et al.* (1997). Europe ambivalent on biotechnology. *Nature*, **387**, 845–7.

# 12 Political risk culture: not just a communication failure

Ian E. Taylor
*Scientific Political Adviser, Greenpeace UK*

## Novartis' genetically modified maize and the continued failure to deal with scientific uncertainty

## Summary

Much has been said about the 'public perception of risk', but it is illuminating to map out the perceptions of risk displayed by those who *use* this phrase, particularly decision-makers. In the food debate at least, comparatively few still perceive the risk debate as purely a data problem. Most have got as far as recognizing 'risk communication' or 'public perception' problems. Many, post-BSE, have gone on to acknowledge that there are structural problems—conflicts of interest and closed processes that need to be replaced by separation of powers and public participation.

However, few appear to have realized the need to shift the risk culture to include 'risk avoidance' where scientific uncertainty is too great and the potential adverse consequences too severe. This judgement requires reframing of the problem to take in the 'big-picture' questions (often value-based) left out by traditional risk assessments but often glaringly obvious to the public. Particularly when the risk makers are not the risk takers and the benefits appear similarly one-sided, policy-makers are unwise to dismiss public views as something to be 'educated out'.

The debate must be reframed to include these valid social, cultural, and environmental positions, and the policy system must take a strongly precautionary approach capable of preventing the risk being generated in the first place, and *able to respond by saying 'no'* to undesirable and unnecessary technological innovations. However, the continuing saga of Ciba-Geigy's (now Novartis') genetically modified maize provides an illustration of how in practice the system currently fails.

# Introduction

## Political misperceptions of risk and science exemplified by food policy

'Open mouth and insert foot' might be offered as an apt summary of politicians' attempts to handle recent fraught issues of food policy by risk communication rather than risk avoidance, the nadir perhaps being former UK Minister of Agriculture John Gummer's misguided attempt to assuage BSE fears by feeding his 4-year old daughter Cordelia a beefburger in a 'photo opportunity'.

Although food policy offers a particularly slippery footing for politicians, their misfortunes here stem from exactly the same misunderstanding about how to handle scientific uncertainty as for many other environmental and health risks. For example, 'no evidence', which in these situations invariably means 'no evidence so far', is construed wrongly as 'no risk'. The BSE crisis in the UK provides abundant examples of this misconstruction. As late as 1994, Minister of Agriculture, Gillian Shephard, said

> 'the Chief Medical Officer continues to advise that there is no evidence whatsoever that BSE causes CJD and, similarly, not the slightest evidence that eating beef or hamburgers causes CJD.' (*Hansard* 1994)

Only two years later, Stephen Dorrell, Secretary of State for Health, referring to 'ten cases of a new variant of CJD' conceded that 'the most likely explanation at present is that these cases are linked to exposure to BSE' (Ministry of Agriculture, Fisheries and Food 1996).

As genetically modified organisms (GMOs) begin to enter the environment and the food chain, the new UK government shows no sign of learning from its predecessor's mistakes and is churning out the same bland reassurances with, apparently, the same failure to comprehend their inadequacy. Jeff Rooker, UK Food Safety Minister, has stated that 'to date, results have not indicated any risks to the agricultural environment from the release of GMOs'. (*Hansard* 1997)

Politicians hope that by shrugging off the responsibility onto technical advisers or committees in this manner they can save themselves from the pitfalls of inevitably inconclusive science. They are sadly oblivious of the fact that if anything the reverse is true, and that to pre-empt trouble they must shoulder their responsibility to lead debate in the cultural-social-political domain, to include the wider issues left out by 'experts'.

Food policy particularly illuminates this dilemma, not least because the presumption that 'technology = progress = good', taken for granted in so many areas where science and policy overlap, falls apart here—despite the best efforts of food technology's proponents to stitch it back together. Is it better to 'interfere' more with food before it reaches the consumer? The minuscule proportion of the market taken by organic produce may belie a potentially greater market. The strategy recently adopted by Tesco, the UK supermarket chain, to price organic produce at the same level as traditional produce suggests a market analysis seeing this as a future growth market worth some loss-leading.

The EU, meanwhile, does not have a sustainable agriculture or food policy. Instead there is the Common Agricultural Policy geared to tackle post-war shortages with its more-cheaper-more-cheaper circle. The public reaction to BSE showed that this production-at-all-costs doctrine can no longer command public support, if indeed it ever could. To quote Sheppard (1997):

'The public were largely unaware, and subsequently shocked to discover, that animal remains were being fed to cattle and were responsible for causing BSE. Such ways of boosting output were beyond public scrutiny. There was an implicit assumption on the part of those who promoted and allowed the practice that the public would broadly support measures which improved productivity. But the subsequent outcry demonstrated that the public rejected the risks of such an 'unnatural' practice. On the contrary, they were horrified that intensive farming methods had been allowed to over-ride and compromise public safety.'

## Views on genetically modified foods

Opinion polls show ambivalence or outright hostility to genetically modified (GM) food. A Europe-wide MORI poll of 4840 people for Greenpeace asked the question: To what extent do you agree or disagree that: 'I personally would be happy to eat genetically modified food?'. 67% were not happy to eat it. A majority of respondents to a recent Eurobarometer survey reported in *Nature* (European Public Concerted Action Group 1997) thought biotechnology in food production should not be encouraged.

Moreover, deeper probing in Unilever-sponsored focus group research indicates a consumer-citizen disjunction that, if it remains unacknowledged, has all the potential to create a public backlash if and when something goes wrong (Grove-White *et al.* 1997). This study revealed a public fatalism that people would have to consume GM food, while nevertheless holding deep reservations. They have no control over the move towards genetic modification of food and no choice but to trust, albeit with suspicion, those who they perceive do control it. So even while *as consumers* they may purchase GM products, if a problem develops then *as citizens* they will expect redress.

This is a worrying conclusion for policy-makers when, over the medium or long term, complex interactions of GM organisms with the environment and the food chain cannot be fully predicted. Professor Philip James, Director of the Rowett Research Institute and author of the Food Standards Agency proposals largely adopted by the UK government, has said of GM foods:

> 'The perception that everything is totally straightforward and safe is utterly naïve. I don't think we understand the dimensions of what we're getting into' (in *Scottish Daily Record* 3rd Feb 1998).

Norman Ellstrand, ecological geneticist at the University of California, has put it very strongly:

> 'within 10 years we will have a moderate to large-scale ecological or economic catastrophe, because there will be so many products being released' (in Kling 1996).

## No way to say 'no'

Set against this backdrop it would seem obvious that the regulatory system should be able to consider options of risk avoidance rather than presume that adverse outcomes will be manageable once a crisis emerges. But the system seems to have no way to say 'no'.

# Novartis' genetically modified maize: a case study

The European marketing approval of Novartis' GM maize ('corn') highlights how, faced with very incomplete scientific knowledge and with virtually no public participation, the distribution of European regulatory power allows imposition of unwanted risks on member states and their citizens—*even when* scientists' reservations about the new technology are as strongly expressed as they are ever likely to be in a debate of this kind.

Only one EU country, France, supported the authorization of Novartis' maize in the European Union. Even France was not sure, and subsequently put a temporary ban on its cultivation in France. The Council of Ministers of the 15 EU countries asked the Commission to withdraw its proposal to approve it. How, then, did it come to be authorized? The answer lies partly in the complex EU decision-making rules and procedures on GMOs, which give most power to the Commission. In particular, under the voting procedures of Directive 90/220/EEC (the 'Deliberate Release Directive') which covers deliberate release into the environment of GMOs, unless member states *unanimously* reject a Commission proposal, the Commissioners can ignore the member states' wishes.

This instance of the EU's 'democratic deficit' is, however, made far worse by misuse of closed scientific committees to provide reassurance of 'no evidence of harm—so far', giving a technical appearance to decisions which in fact are driven by US-backed commercial pressure. The consequence is that decision-makers escape with no accountability for their decisions, without having to justify the real grounds for their decisions, or why they ignore the 'big-picture' questions.

## The GM maize itself—what is it and why is it contentious?

Ciba Geigy (now merged with Sandoz to form Novartis) has genetically modified a maize to contain three bacterial genes that produce:

- resistance to the herbicide Basta (glufosinate ammonium)
- a bacillus thuringiensis (Bt) 'cry' toxin to kill the European corn borer pest
- antibiotic (ampicillin) resistance, a 'marker' gene used in laboratory tests when developing the maize.

The most major concern has been around the antibiotic resistance gene, which in fact Novartis could have removed from the final product. The opposition here derives from concern that this could transfer to harmful bacteria in the gut of animals and humans, compromising the use of a valuable family of antibiotics.[1] There is also concern at the Bt gene, both regarding possible adverse effects on beneficial insects, and regarding its capacity to rapidly generate Bt resistance in the pest insect population, thereby threatening the existing use of a less active form of Bt in spray form by organic farmers.[2]

The herbicide resistance property is also contentious. Concern centres around how this sets a trend towards wider use of a 'broad spectrum' herbicide which kills all foliage upon contact. In the centre of origin of maize (Central and South America); there is also the worry that this gene will cross-pollinate into weedy relatives creating herbicide-resistant 'super weeds'.

---

1. A letter to the UK Department of the Environment from the Ministry of Agriculture, Fisheries and Food (MAFF) Biotechnology Unit dated 15 May 1995 states that 'members [of the Advisory Committee on Novel Foods and Processes] were concerned that clearance of the unprocessed GM maize would condone "sloppy" genetic modification.' The *New Scientist*, 4 January 1997, notes that Professor John Beringer, Head of the UK Advisory Committee on Releases to the Environment (ACRE) was ' "staggered" that Ciba did not avoid the controversy by removing the beta-lactamase gene from the maize before applying to market it'.
2. These concerns were the basis of a petition initiating legal action against the US Environmental Protection Agency lodged on 16 September 1997 by 31 groups including Green-peace, the International Federation of Organic Agriculture Movements, the Sierra Club, the Centre for International Technology Assessment in Washington, the Institute for Agriculture and Trade Policy in Minneapolis, and the National Coalition for Mis-use of Pesticide.

Further concerns derive from unknown allergenic or other adverse effects from all these genes, which have never before been part of the food chain.

## The saga up to June 1998: a blow-by-blow account

In 1994 Ciba Geigy gave its scientific dossier on Bt maize to the French government for consideration. Almost all that data was from the company's own experiments, and it omitted some negative data which Ciba Geigy earlier submitted to US authorities (e.g. that the Bt maize can harm beneficial organisms[3]). The detailed chronology of events then ran as follows:

### March 1995

France passed the dossier and decision-making to the European Commission for application under Directive 90/220/EEC.

### April 1996

The European Commission proposed the maize to the so-called 'Article 21' committee, made up of civil servants representing the member states. Many, due to advice from their own scientific advisors, were doubtful. The vote was:

Opposed—UK, Denmark, Austria, Sweden

Abstained—Luxembourg, Greece, Germany, Italy

Supported—Finland, Ireland, Belgium, Portugal, Spain

Invalid vote—Netherlands (approved, but not for human food).

This did not constitute a qualified majority needed to approve the Commission's recommendation. Under the rules, the Commission could then take the decision-making to the Council of Ministers (that is, the Environment Ministers of the 15 member states).

Some of those opposed, for example the UK's Advisory Committee on Novel Foods and Processes (ACNFP), took a sophisticated perspective of the nature of the risk. Its then chair, Professor Derek Burke commented 'We decided that although the technical risk was small, the consequential risk

---

3. In a letter to the Department of the Environment dated 19 May, the MAFF Biotechnology Unit complains that 'The maize contains an intact bla gene which encodes B-lactamase, an enzyme which rapidly degrades penicillin-type antibiotics. This gene has a bacterial promoter. Its presence in the maize was not included in the description of the GMO and minimal reference was made to it in the notification.' This letter also requests the Department of the Environment to advise the European Commission that 'we have a serious concern' and to 'raise an objection to the granting of a consent'.

could be very large'.[4] Another member of the same committee has since spelt it out more strongly:[5]

> 'my principal fear is that, if you take this material and feed it unprocessed—particularly unprocessed—to an animal, or indeed, even a human being, what will happen is that eventually—because of the length of time of contact of the DNA in the system—you will get transformation of an E. coli or an enterobacter in the intestine. Once you have done that, you will get a high-level antibiotic resistance, a kind of resistance which will take apart a dose of ampicillin in less than 30 minutes. We're already in an era when antibiotics are a problem. We do not have sufficient antibiotics and antibiotic resistance is increasing dramatically in a number of micro-organisms. I do not believe that we should be pushing the boundaries even further by introducing this kind of problem.'

As it turns out, this eminently sensible approach was not going to prevail over the Commission.

## 25 June 1996

The Council of Ministers met. Only France was in favour, Spain undecided. The 13 other states, including the UK, did not want the Bt maize for various reasons. The Council decided not to vote on the proposal and asked the Commission to withdraw it. By not voting, the Council was considered to have 'not acted', even though it asked for the withdrawal of the proposal. Directive 90/220/EEC says that a proposal from the Commission must be adopted within three months 'if the Council has not acted'.

Why didn't the 15 ministers vote in the Council? The vote would have been 13 against, one in favour, and one abstention. Again, they would have 'not acted' to approve the Commission's proposal (which only requires a qualified majority), and 'not acted' to unanimously reject it. The maize would therefore have received authorization. By refusing to vote and demanding that the Commission withdraw the proposed authorization, the Council was hoping to use its political power outside the committee rules to stop the maize.

---

4. 19th Annual Campden Day Lecture, 4 June 1997. See also Professor Burke's comments in Chapter 11 above, which reflect other noteworthy points made in the lecture. The French Comite de la Prevention et de la Precaution (CPP) opinion of 5 September 1997 makes a similar point 'Il est souligne que la notion de rarete d'un evenement de transfert de gene n'est pas suffisante pour en faire un argument rassurant. En effect, chez les bacteries, dans la nature, les transferts de genes sont extremement nombreux'. ('We would emphasize that saying that a gene transfer event is rare is not, of itself, a reassuring argument. In fact, transfers of genes are extremely numerous amongst bacteria in the natural environment.') [translation by Greenpeace]. It goes on to recommend prohibition of GM plants containing antibiotic resistance genes.
5. Professor Tony Atkinson, *Newsnight* BBC2 TV, 13 January 1998. Professor Atkinson had also noted that, a propos the antibiotic resistance gene 'No one has yet looked at the effect of feeding a gene to lots of animals day in day out for years' (*New Scientist*, 4 January 1997, p. 8).

'Only one country, France, supported the position [to approve the maize] and even they were wavering' a Commission spokesman told reporters. 'The rest said, for different reasons, withdraw it or reconsider it.' (Reuters 26 June 1996)

Far from withdrawing the proposal, the Commission then 'consulted' its own scientific committees, with very narrow terms of reference. For example, the Scientific Committee for Animal Nutrition (SCAN) was asked 'to confirm that there is no reason to believe that the genetic modification of the maize will give rise to any adverse effects on animal health'.

## 18 December

After considering the opinions of those scientific committees, the Commission decided to authorize the import and cultivation of the maize.

Leaked minutes of the discussions revealed that the fear of 'trade problems' with the USA had influenced the approval:

'Sir Leon Brittan [Commission Vice-President] supports the proposal ... which as he emphasises, will make relations with the US easier ... Mrs Bonino [Commissioner for Consumer Policy] says she believes that the decision is taken because of economic pressure ... [and regretted that] the Commission had to take a decision on an issue about which the public feels so strongly, under pressure and urged on because of the import of considerable stocks of maize from the US'

(Minutes of Commission meeting 18 December 1997
as published in *Le Soir*).

The Commission press release of this date, however, frames the issue entirely in terms of the science. Moreover it uses a highly simplistic phraseology regarding the nature of the risk:

'There is no reason to believe that the genetic modification of the Bt maize will give rise to any adverse effects on human health from its use in human food. There is no reason to believe that the genetic modification of the Bt maize will give rise to any adverse effects on animal health from its use in animal feed'.

Presumably the intention was to give an impression of certainty where none exists, but after BSE reassurances cast in identical terms this seems likely to have the opposite effect, if anything raising public suspicions.

## 23 January 1997

The European Commission officially adopted its proposal to approve the maize.

## 4 February 1997

France gave official authorization for the GM maize and notified all other

EU Member States. From this point onwards, the maize could legally be marketed throughout the EU.

## 8/9 February 1997

Austria and Luxembourg announced a temporary ban on the maize, under Article 16 of 90/220/EEC. This reads:

> 'Where a Member State has justifiable reasons to consider that a product which has been properly notified and has received written consent under this Directive constitutes a risk to human health or the environment, it may provisionally restrict or prohibit the use and/or sale of that product on its territory'.

Argument immediately ensued over 'justifiable reasons' which the Commission interprets to mean 'new information'.

## 12 February 1997

French Prime Minister, Alain Juppe, announced that cultivation of the maize would not be allowed in France for ecological reasons. Axel Kahn, the chairman of the Commission du Genie Biomoleculaire (CGB), the competent authority for France, promptly resigned. The remarkable situation from this point on was that no member state could properly be said to be in favour of the maize, which nevertheless has cleared the official EU regulatory process.

## March 1997

Italy used Article 16 to temporarily ban its cultivation in Italy.

## April 1997

The European parliament voted 407 to 2 to demand that authorization be suspended. This vote carried no official weight.

1.2 million Austrians (from a total electorate of 5.8 million) endorsed the Austrian ban on the maize by supporting a referendum against all GM food or release of GMOs in Austria. Austrian referenda operate like petitions, not on a yes/no vote basis. This was the second highest ever number of signatories and the biggest ever on an environmental issue.

US government and industry lobbying pressure increased, including meetings between Commission officials and the US Department of Agriculture.

## 14 May 1997

According to Directive 90/220/EEC procedures, this was the deadline for a decision whether to allow Austria to maintain its ban: the 'Article 21

Committee' of member states' 'competent authorities' should have met and decided by this date. The Commission allowed the deadline to slip past, apparently hoping that the issue would cool off. It took the position that such bans should not be allowed, having once again consulted its scientific committees.

The rules for this decision then followed the same pattern as before. Adoption of the Commission's proposal to disallow Austria's ban would require a qualified majority. For all other votes, including unanimity against the Commission, the decision would be referred to the Council of Ministers.

## 22 September 1997
Italy decided to lift its Article 16 ban on maize cultivation.

## 5 November 1997
The Article 21 Committee met and discussed the maize, but the Commission acceded to Austrian and Luxembourg requests for a postponement of the vote when it became apparent that it would not get support by the necessary qualified majority. It appears that at least Austria, Belgium, Denmark, Ireland, Luxembourg, Sweden, and the UK would not have supported the Commission.

## 12 November 1997
The first shipment of the US autumn harvest of maize arrived and was blockaded in Rotterdam by Greenpeace, who not only objected to the Novartis maize but pointed out that several other GM varieties grown in the US but not legally approved for sale in Europe were probably mixed in.

## 27 November 1997
France reversed its position and announced that it would allow cultivation of maize. Apparently as a sort of public palliative, however, it also made the contradictory announcement that it would prevent planting of other GM crops[6] pending public debate, and would not vote against Austria's Article 16 ban!

## 8 January 1998
About 100 farmers from the second-largest French farmers union, Confederation Paysanne, attacked a Novartis' conditioning and storage plant.

---

6. Remarkably, the French Comite de la Prevention et de la Precaution (CPP) issued a public correction (CPP, 4th December 1997) to the interpretation of their position in the Prime Minister's press release: 'The experts present did, however, emphasise the possibility of risks of inter-species transfer of marker genes used for selection of transgenic varieties and, notably, genes for resistance to antibiotics. They particularly recommend that all varieties of crops with a transgenic configuration containing an antibiotic marker should not be allowed on the market (the Novartis maize variety does, however, contain such a marker).' [translation by Greenpeace]

They found 5 tons of GM maize, which they destroyed. Three of their representatives were arrested.

## 9 January 1998

The Article 21 Committee met and again failed to vote after the Commission agreed to a further delay, probably because France had now joined those opposed.

## 15 April 1998

In a postal vote of Article 21 Committee members, the European Commission failed to get sufficient support to outlaw Austria and Luxembourg's bans. This meant that the decision would have to go to the Council of EU Environment Ministers.

## May 1998

In the meantime, the wisdom of allowing cultivation of the maize was further questioned by new findings that two-thirds of the larvae of lacewings, a beneficial predator insect, died when fed corn borer pests that had fed on the maize (Hilbeck et al. 1998). The Bt toxin had been predicted not to have this kind of effect.

In June 1998, the EU Environment Ministers will meet and may take a decision on the bans. However, as with the authorization itself, if the Commission insists on opposing Austria and Luxembourg, the procedure requires unanimity of member states to overrule the Commission. In the last resort, Austria has indicated it will take the issue to the European Court of Justice.[7]

# Commentary

## Decision-makers' analysis of risk

In extracting lessons from this case it is illuminating to map out the perceptions of risk displayed by decision-makers. Much has been said and

---

7. As this article goes to press, the saga continues. EU Environment Ministers chose not to vote at their June 1998 meeting and had failed to act by the deadline of September 1998. The Commission is therefore allowed to adopt its position and announce that Austria and Luxembourg have acted illegally, but so far they have chosen not to. Meanwhile, in September 1998, the highest French administrative court, the Conseil d'Etat, upheld a legal suit by Greenpeace that the authorization documentation from Novartis was incomplete regarding long-term effects of the antibiotic resistance gene on human health, and withdrew the governmental permit to grow Novartis maize in France. In December 1998 the Conseil d'Etat then referred the matter to the European Court of Justice to decide whether this unilateral ban action was legal under EU rules, triggering a protracted legal process with the immediate effect that the maize cannot be planted in France in 1999.

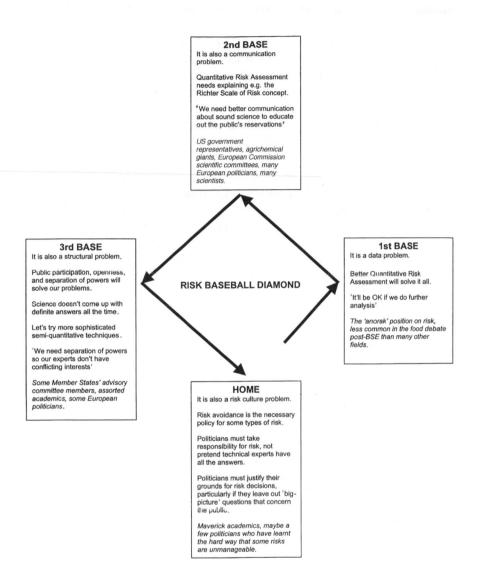

**Fig. 12.1** Risk Baseball Diamond—schematic of decision-makers' positions on risks to health and environment, particularly for genetically modified foods. Two related parameters increase round the diamond: 1) decision-makers' recognition of inevitable scientific uncertainty, 2) decision-makers' recognition that this can only be resolved by reframing the debate to include other non-technical factors (e.g. values).

written about the 'public perception of risk': indeed it is a favourite phrase of politicians keen to brush away reaction to an unpopular decision by casting the public as irrational or unreasonable. But what about the *political* perception of risk? What is the view if we turn around the telescope and look at decision-makers' views of risk—not just of elected politicians themselves, but also of the policy community, including government employees and expert advisory bodies?

While decision-makers display a continuum of risk viewpoints, certain sets of arguments appear repeatedly and can be roughly grouped together. Figure 12.1 offers a schematic categorization of positions in the form of a 'Risk Baseball Diamond'. Lest baseball aficionados imagine unintended subtleties of significance, this is simply a means to visualize the state of the debate. Some players are strung out between bases, and the shape should not be taken to suggest repeated circular motion—there is a progression towards 'home base' as a position defining an environmentally acceptable view of risk. It should also be noted that the type of risk under considera-tion is that characterized by scientific uncertainty, potentially widespread, irreversible and severe impact, and probably also long lead-times and in-voluntary exposure. Although the schematic makes particular reference to the GM food debate, its applicability is intended to be wider.

In the food debate at least, comparatively few decision-makers still perceive the risk debate as purely a data problem (1st base).

Most have got as far as recognizing the 'risk communication' or 'public perception of risk' problems (2nd base).

Many have acknowledged that there is a structural problem (3rd base): that conflicts of interest and closed processes need to be replaced by separation of powers and public participation in decisions.

Very few have realized that it is also necessary to shift the risk culture to include 'risk avoidance' (home base) because, for some categories of risk, scientific uncertainty is too great and the potential adverse consequences too severe. This judgement requires reframing the problem to take in the 'big-picture' questions.

So, in progressing around the diamond, two related parameters in-crease:

> decision-makers' recognition of the inevitability of scientific uncertainty for some sorts of important risk debates (here, the impacts of GM foods on health and the environment);

> recognition that this necessitates reframing the debate to reach a resolution by including broader, often non-technical considerations (like 'does society want GM food?', 'what level of risk from GMOs released into the environment is acceptable, *if any*?').

## Positions adopted in the maize debate

The US government officials and the agrichemical giants generating GM foods appear to have the shallowest comprehension of the scientific uncertainties and the validity of arguments arising from them.[8] So far as they are concerned, European consumers are ignorant and the problem can either be 'educated out' or they should be ignored on the grounds that they will come round once they find they have unwillingly or unwittingly been eating GM foods. They are completely stuck at base two, at least as regards their public statements (arguably some have not even got beyond first base!). The power relationship and the level of domestic resistance is such that the US sees no necessity to give it more thought. This, of course, offers it an apparently simple route to promote its agribusiness, but ironically, because this has led to a European perception that they being are force-fed GM foods, a deeper understanding of the risk might have served its longer-term interests better.

Many European scientists share the viewpoint that it is essentially a presentational issue, as does much of government, exemplified perhaps by the establishment of bodies with names like 'Risk Communication Unit' (a joint body between the UK Ministry of Agriculture, Fisheries and Food and the Department of Health recently formed specifically to handle food risks). The European Commission scientific committees' position in the press release announcing approval of the maize (quoted earlier) shows zero recognition of the large domain of scientific ignorance associated with GM maize. As a result its reassurances sound bland and unconvincing.

At points in the maize saga, various member states' advisory bodies show themselves to have got beyond this, to base 3. Their view of the ampicillin resistance risk at least notes the potential extent and significance of the bad-case scenario, and shows some recognition of important scientific uncertainties. Some of these committees do include consumer representation, although it is unclear how much that is responsible for this difference in stance. In setting up bodies like the UK's embryo Food Standards Agency there is a search for more open mechanisms with better linkages to the broader public, and a de-linkage from food industry vested interests. This reflects a dawning recognition by some politicians that the best scientific advice does have its limitations, and that—if only to save their own skins— they need processes with greater democratic legitimacy. The European Commission did make one step towards 3rd base in 1997 with the recognition

---

8. For example, US Agriculture Secretary Dan Glickman has said (regarding GM soya) that objections to GM crops are mainly irrational and 'as long as they do prove safe, science must prevail over emotion when it comes to our trade rules' (Reuters, 3 December 1997).

of the need for structural change to 'separate powers'. This led to the transfer of its scientific advisory committees on food matters to a new home in the Directorate-General responsible for Consumer Policy and Health Protection.

That is where progress, at least in official circles, largely stops. Calls for a complete change to the risk culture, bringing in 'big-picture' questions about whether the risk is justifiable, are only heard from outside the establishment. Indeed, with the Deliberate Release Directive 90/220/EEC up for review, the pressure from the Commission has been to push for a 'streamlining' of procedures and an even greater reliance on risk assessment, a narrowly defined case-by-case technical approach that utterly fails to address the most fundamental questions. It omits, for example, questions of precedent-setting, or of the justification for imposing a GM food risk on the population, or of the cumulative impacts on the population or the environment of lots of GM food and crops.

## Opening up the debate

Even where consumer representatives sit on committees like the UK's Advisory Committee on Releases to the Environment (ACRE), or the Advisory Committee on Novel Foods and Processes (ACNFP), the scope of the debate has very largely been restricted to a case-by-case discussion of the technical merits of each application. Proper consumer representation, drawing on what is known about public opinion, would point to the need for a fundamental challenge to the desirability of *any* GMOs in food or the environment.

There is, however, no sign that consumer representatives on these committees have succeeded in opening this debate. This might in part be due to narrowly drawn terms of reference, but it is also clear that these representatives are in a small minority and face an uphill task to prevail against the dominant mindset—assuming that they don't share it themselves. As Sheppard (1997) puts it:

> 'There is, for example, a widespread and 'taken-for-granted' assumption in the regulatory community that GM technology is the basis for future economic growth and international competitiveness and is therefore desirable. Those with the necessary qualifications to advise governments on the risks tend to be already working actively in the field of gene technology, whether in academic institutions or companies. This makes them both the best and the worst judges. Whilst the assessment benefits from their expertise and experience it is also likely to be blinkered by their inability to question the underlying assumptions of genetic modification.'

Consumer representatives are also in the exposed position of trying to argue that our ignorance of what might happen is too great to press ahead. By definition, nothing is known of areas of ignorance beyond the reach of scientific prediction, and this situation is rarely remedied since funding is not readily forthcoming for research that might expose good reasons not to push ahead with profitable new biotechnologies. In contrast, the arguments to press ahead are backed by a tonnage of data.

One of the striking aspects of the maize case is that expert committees have nevertheless expressed disapproval in forthright terms (e.g. the ACNFP[9]). However, commercial-political pressure, combined with the democratic deficit in European decision-making, has been able to force it onto the market anyway.[10] Scientific committees at the European level were misused to generate a 'no evidence = no risk' argument and disallow opposition. It was the opposition who effectively carried the burden of proof, despite the supposed presumption of precaution in the preamble to the relevant EU Directive:

> '... action by the Community relating to the environment should be based on the principle that preventive action should be taken' (Council Directive 90/220 1990).

## Risk avoidance

Risk avoidance (with its correlative, risk elimination) is usually not even considered as an alternative to risk management—or rather, for issues likeGMOs, *the pretence that there can be* risk management. But it is the onlysensible approach for certain categories of risk. In this respect it isencouraging to note the recent Department of Health decision that 'precautionary advice is warranted' to avoid mercury amalgam fillings during pregnancy *despite* finding 'no evidence of harm to children' on the basis of the 'possibility that mercury vapour emitted during the removal or insertion of amalgam during dental treatment could cross the placenta' (Department of Health 1998). To be effective, precautionary action must necessarily be taken in advance of conclusive evidence. Waiting for final evidence means the precautionary options left open are then far more drastic

---

9. 'The ACNFP considered that any risk of transfer of this bla gene and its associated bacterial regulatory sequences however low was unacceptable', ACNFP, Report on Processed Products from Genetically-Modified (GM) Insect-Resistant Maize, May 1996.
10. The present proposals to revise the Deliberate Release Directive seem to recognize that changes to the voting procedures are needed, but it is far from evident that this will ensure sufficient balance and it will do nothing to deal with the other issues raised here about misuse of scientific advice.

and draconian, like banning beef on the bone just as the BSE saga finally appears to be entering its closing stages.

When it comes to food, it is quite rational for a member of the public to decide that they do not want *any* pesticide residues, or *any* BSE prions, or *any* GM organisms. Such a position cannot be invalidated by more or better expert advice. It is, after all, quite possible to have food production systems which avoid all of these. Even for problems that are arguably more integral to food production and hence less amenable to risk avoidance, there are good examples of this approach. After an outbreak of salmonella which killed 100 people in 1952, Sweden embarked on a long-term policy to eliminate it from the food chain. Salmonella prevalence is now at less than 1%. UK figures for poultry show that one-third are contaminated with significant pathogens, although salmonella accounts for only a proportion of that figure (Lang *et al.* 1997).

To take another controversy over GM food, many consumer organizations have been calling for the segregation of Monsanto's GM 'Roundup Ready' soya, but so far in vain. Despite the protestations of agribusiness to the contrary, segregation is of course quite feasible. Monsanto's and other firms' arguments that segregation would be too expensive are, of course, predicated on the assumption that GM will take over and a single non-segregated stream will be fine in the long run. But at the moment consumer resistance in Europe is such that GM-free soya supplies are achieving a price premium. It is both ironic and unfair that retailers wishing to source the traditional product should have to bear the extra costs, rather than these costs attaching to the novel product and Monsanto. But Monsanto is in a position to use its market power to pursue a 'force-feeding' policy which it believes will return the quickest, biggest profits.

## Final comments

As with many other environmental/technological risks, the risk makers (in this case agrichemical companies) are not the risk takers (in this case consumers). The benefits appear similarly one-sided. The justification of the technology, cast in terms of money-economy-jobs, takes no account of the external costs accrued by the risk takers. There is no explicit balancing of the risks and benefits viewed from any perspective other than that of agribusiness. Nor is there any attempt to consider the costs of a 'backlash' to farmers, or the Treasury, or the environmental costs of a bad-case or worst-case genetic release problem.

Policy-makers are inclined to dismiss adverse public response as based on 'dread' or 'ignorance'. But they are unwary if they choose to dismiss public views about GM foods as fears to be 'educated out'. If a problem arises, the public, having been ignored, are democratically entitled to complain. This kind of backlash carries moral authority, which is why it is so politically lethal.

To avoid the political risks from environmental and health risks like GMOs, decision-makers need to be bold enough to accept their responsibility to lead the debate at the outset and justify which issues are included and which left out.

## REFERENCES

Council Directive (1990). *Official Journal of the European Communities* (Directive 90/220/EEC), 8 May, No L 117/17.

Department of Health (1998). Press release, 29 April 1998. See also web site http://www.coi.gov.uk/coi/depts/GDH/coi0929e.ok

European Public Concerted Action Group (1997). Europe ambivalent on biotechnology. *Nature*, **387**, 845–7.

Grove-White, R., Macnaghten, P., Mayer, S., and Wynne, B. (1997). *Uncertain world: genetically modified organisms, food and public attitudes in Britain*. Centre for the Study of Environmental Change in association with Unilever, Lancaster University.

*Hansard* (1994). Parliamentary written answer to PQ 1723, 30 June.

*Hansard* (1997). Parliamentary written answer tp PQ, 25 June.

Hilbeck, A., Baumgartner, M., Fried, P. M., and Bigler, F. (1998). Effects of transgenic Bacillus thuringiensis corn-fed prey on mortality and development time of immature Chrysoperla carnea (Neuroptera: Chrysopidae). *Environmental Entomology*, **27**, 480–7.

Kling, J. (1996). Could transgenic crops one day breed superweeds? *Science*, **274**, 180–1.

Lang, T., Millstone, E., and Rayner, M. (1997). *Food standards and the state: a fresh start*, (Discussion paper 3). Centre for Food Policy, Thames Valley University.

Ministry of Agriculture, Fisheries and Food (1996). *Food Safety Information Bulletin*, April 1996. Ministry of Agriculture Fisheries and Food, London.

Sheppard, J. (1997). *From BSE to genetically modified organisms: science, uncertaintyand the precautionary principle*. Report for Greenpeace.

# 13 Consumers and risk

Sheila McKechnie and Sue Davies
*Consumers' Association*

## Introduction

Since its inception, the Consumers' Association (CA) has been involved in the evaluation and communication of risk. In its early years its work concentrated on the safety of domestic appliances but as consumer needs have changed, the CA has sought to meet demands for information on risk on everything from the Channel Tunnel to BSE. We are, therefore, an alternative source of information on risk and a participant in the wider social and political process of determining risk and establishing an appropriate level of safety. This paper is based on our own experience of the information needs of consumers and of the wider system. It draws mainly on our experiences within the food policy area, but our conclusions will have broader implications.

## The wider environment

Our first proposition is simple. Governmental bodies and other quangos charged with assessing risk and recommending action are out of touch with the changed environment in which they are operating. Politicians who talk about modernizing government are usually referring to national and local government institutions and the process of elections. However, the decisions that impact directly on people are often taken in the hidden substructure of committees, quangos, and unaccountable bodies that few understand and even fewer have access to. The following analysis of the gaps in the system applies to government mechanisms as a whole, but has specific relevance to the control of risk.

### Decline in deference

Decision-making by experts or the 'great and the good' behind closed doors, resulting in the pronouncements of decisions without explanation, has come under serious attack from individuals and organizations who regard such attitudes as patronizing and inadequate. But for reasons that can be debated, we no longer automatically defer to authority in any of its forms (Consumers' Association, Sainsbury's and Unilever 1998).

Individual experts often react badly to challenges to their knowledge and decisions, without understanding that it is not what they do or have done, but the process that confers such rights that is under challenge. Decisions are all too often presented as though they are backed up by relatively conclusive science when this is often not the case. The committees within which these experts operate in general have narrow technical remits. Without any other mechanism for considering broader issues, the social context in which they are deliberating frequently gets missed. The problem of the narrow mandates of these committees and decision-making bodies is not unique to the UK—it applies globally. The result is that the real questions that need to be debated rarely get a hearing.

The decline in deference not only applies to the scientist, but also to government. Consumers are now less likely to defer to government pronouncements about risk. A CA survey carried out just after the announcement of a possible link between BSE and CJD showed that 71% of consumers believed that the government had withheld information about the risks associated with BSE (Davies and Todd 1996). Only 21% agreed that overall they were 'confident in the advice that the government provides on the safety of the food we eat'. When asked to rank according to sources of impartial advice about food safety, the government was ranked below the food industry (see Table 13.1). The closed system in which such decisions were being made only helped to fuel this scepticism. This survey was repeated in relation to BSE advice in October 1998. Little had changed, with Government advice still rated below the food industry (Consumers' Association 1999).

## Expert decision-making

A number of factors have reduced confidence in the objectivity of science and raised questions about its limitations. The concept of 'mandated' expertise has had low recognition in Britain, where there has been a tendency to assume that science itself is independent, irrespective of who is expressing a view. As pointed out in previous chapters, however, this is now under serious challenge.

We are also increasingly faced with the problem that expertise in some areas will lie predominantly with industry. The research, for example in relation to new food technologies, will often have been undertaken to achieve commercial objectives. There is the danger that developments will progress before we have answered some of the more basic, fundamental questions that relate to public health. It is therefore essential that we develop ways of

**Table 13.1**   Trusted sources of impartial advice

| Source | Most trustworthy (%) | Least trustworthy (%) |
|---|---|---|
| Health professionals (e.g. GPs, health visitors) | 36 | 3 |
| Consumer organizations (e.g. National Consumer Council, Consumers' Association) | 27 | 4 |
| Scientists specializing in food safety | 20 | 5 |
| Government departments | 5 | 49 |
| The food industry | 5 | 30 |
| Don't know | 8 | 9 |

(2021 adults aged over 15, representative of all adults in Great Britain, were interviewed in their homes between 19 and 23 April 1996. Source: Consumers' Association 1996.)

ensuring that there is still an independent science base within the UK and that independent scientific experts are available to advise the government.

If we are to re-establish trust in these institutions, we need to tackle this problem of independence. Full declaration of all relevant interests is fundamental. The need for a multidisciplinary approach is also essential. As the BSE crisis has demonstrated, there was no public health expert on the Spongiform Encephalopathy Advisory Committee, which advises the government on BSE, until December 1995—reliance on a narrow range of scientific disciplines fails to address broader issues.

## Limitations of science

Science itself is also under attack, a victim of its own promotion. Many developments and innovations have proved two-edged. It is no accident that the issue of food exposes this debate most starkly. The methods used to produce food have become increasingly complex. Many consumers feel in some unspecific way that they want more 'natural' food, whereas industry sees new technologies such as genetic modification as the way to produce safer, higher quality, and more nutritious food. People see science and technology in this context as having produced the current food safety and health problems and are cynical therefore about the application of science as providing a solution. BSE has fuelled this concern. It is often the case that the public can see few direct benefits for themselves in new food technology (Consumers' Association 1997), yet feel that ultimately they are the ones being asked to take the risks. Debates on food safety are likely, therefore, to be characterized by some of the most extreme and fundamental rejections of the view of science as progress. Social, ethical, and moral objections to the way that developments are leading has made many consumers increasingly wary. A MORI survey commissioned by the Government on public attitudes to risk, for example, found that 53% of respondents wanted more legislation on genetically-modified foods (MORI 1999). Some are likely to take the view that science has got it wrong. Given this, trying to create an institutional structure for decision-making in this sector is likely to be very difficult.

It is important to be clear that we are not advocating that there is no place for sound science, we simply need to be more aware of its limitations (Sheppard 1998). Science will always be needed to inform policy decisions. The danger comes in overestimating the role that it can play. The public has become tired of false reassurances of safety and of decisions presented as though they are relatively conclusive when fundamental uncertainties still remain. It is naive to assume that a pure science approach can ever be taken (Consumers' Association 1999). Recent experiences, for example, in relation to the use of antibiotic-resistant marker genes in genetically modified crops, have highlighted how different scientific committees within the UK and the European Union can reach different conclusions, based on the same evidence (see Chapter 12; Advisory Committee on Novel Food and Processes 1995; Scientific Committee for Animal Nutrition 1996; Scientific Committee for Food 1996). Their decisions differed according to whether or not they felt that the risk posed was an acceptable one to take. Scientists regularly have to make value judgements that can have huge ramifications for society, although their pronouncements will often be clouded by scientific justification. Decisions will often be a matter of best expert judgement—the advice of scientists, rather than 'scientific advice'.

## Access to information

The closed systems of decision-making described above depend largely on the control of, and access to, information. Such information historically has been difficult to obtain and therefore the views of experts difficult to challenge. This is no longer the case. Many people now have access to the Internet. It is possible for anyone with a modem link and a computer to access vast amounts of information. Any expert, or indeed anyone who dissents from a particular judgement on risk, can set up a web site and make their views known. Regulatory bodies themselves can, at very low cost, provide vast quantities of information that would simply have been too expensive in old paper-based technologies.

One of the problems with this information revolution is that there is often little to identify the credibility or otherwise of the source. Views that have little or no basis in scientific research are often posited against substantive research-based opinions as if they were equal in weight, when this is clearly not the case. It can therefore often be difficult to get a clear picture of the state of the evidence. The essential point, however, is that we are all experts now—or think we are.

At the same time that this revolution has been taking place, government decision-making has all too often remained behind closed doors. It has been difficult to find out the basis of government policy decisions and to be clear about their motivations. Information has been classified as commercially confidential without any clear justification, and it has been virtually impossible to obtain copies of the evidence considered by scientific advisory committees as well as the uncertainties and assumptions involved in their deliberations. There has also been a failure to give credence to minority scientific opinion. The obvious example is again BSE, where despite an enormous amount of uncertainty, there was a failure to acknowledge the possibility of a link with CJD until several years later (see Chapter 7). Policy was based on limited evidence that BSE would follow the scrapie model. Attempts to suppress such opinions, rather than addressing them within the context of a broader public debate, only serve to undermine trust. Attempts to open up the advisory committee structure are now being put in place, but still need to go further.

# The changing nature of risk

Food and health scares have often been dismissed as media hype. So, does the media create fears about risks or simply reflect the nature of risks in modern society? As the statement 'x is not a risk' is usually not considered news, the media must, by its nature, create a climate of exaggeration about risk. The sheer availability of information through print and broadcast media also has its own dynamic. While the government sits on information used in its own deliberations, the media will continue to set the agenda.

But it is also the case that the nature of risk is changing in modern society, e.g. patterns of disease have changed significantly this century. Risks that were not foreseen and certainly not managed have inflicted a heavy toll, for example AIDS. It is all too often the unintended consequences of change that create problems. They are also incredibly difficult to predict. No one has suggested that the food industry has deliberately exposed the population to risks from BSE, but changes in practices have had consequences that were not foreseen. In the debate about genetically modified foods, few are saying that current developments will have adverse effects on human health or the environment. Most are saying that we simply don't know.

## The traditional approach

Traditionally—as noted in Chaper 12—there has been a case-by-case approach to assessing potential risks. While this may be appropriate for evaluation of specific chemicals, for example, the same approach can not be adopted for issues that have a broader social context (Stern and Fineberg 1996). In the case of genetically modified foods, approval has been carried out on this case-by-case basis. Substantial equivalence is the principle upon which safety is based—comparing a new product with what is already known about an existing one. But technological developments such as this may bring with them ethical, moral, and religious dilemmas. Their short-term impact needs to be considered in relation to the long-term costs on the environment and on public health. The potential consequences would be enormous if we were to get it wrong, as genetically modified ingredients are already present in a vast number of products. There therefore needs to be a mechanism for considering the consequences of the technology as a whole, and its broader impact, as a wide range of genetically modified products go on the market.

## Social acceptability

The major dilemma that we need to tackle is how to achieve a level of risk that is socially acceptable when we may not have all of the facts to hand to enable a proper and accurate assessment of the risk. While we are moving towards a more inclusive system of decision-making and accepting that science alone is not a sufficient basis for decision-making where outcomes are political, social, and economic, there needs to be greater debate within science itself about the need for a radical change in the way we approach risk. While it is the case that the Health and Safety Commission (HSC) has done much within the field of occupational risk analysis to develop approaches that formulate risk characterizations in a theoretical way, much input into other decision-making structures has remained profoundly empiricist. We need to find a way of balancing the limitations of an empiricist approach with broader socio-economic input.

## The precautionary principle

As we have discussed, it may not always be possible to quantify clearly what the long-term costs and benefits of new developments will be. Despite this, technological change is taking place at a rapid pace. This is not necessarily a negative development—it can offer benefits and opportunities; but it also means that much of the research has been based on addressing commercial needs. We now need to frame the questions correctly from the beginning—before there is no going back. If the research doesn't give us a clear picture we should delay a decision until the research can provide us with a clearer picture. In effect, this means ensuring the precautionary approach.

But if in any risk decision-making process the level of proof required for action is causal and verifiable, then this itself acts as the barrier to the implementation of the precautionary principle. At the other extreme, if we take all potential or theoretical outcomes as likely to happen then innovation would be stifled. Current attempts to quantify the risks that are likely from the amount of BSE that has gone into the human food chain have stumbled on this problem. If you take the most pessimistic assumptions, the number of human cases of nv CJD could be up to half the population. If you take very optimistic assumptions, only a few cases will arise. Decision-making in such a context becomes difficult and the science will be of only limited help. Risk assessment cannot be understood as a strictly scientific approach—we need to adapt it to ensure that broader societal issues can be addressed from the outset.

# Individualism and regulation

## Personal choice

However it is explained or described, part of the rejection of 'closed' decision-making is the belief that we have the right to make our own decisions. Where the risk at issue is one that entirely relates to the individual and has no social, economic, or political consequences then the individual should decide. Very few risks, however, come into this category, as most involve complex and inter-related social, economic, and political factors.

Allowing individual consumers to choose for themselves whether or not to take action, based on whether or not they consider there to be a risk or benefit for themselves, may have consequences for future generations. The question then becomes not one of what is to be decided but who is to make the decision. The legitimacy of the structure is then open to challenge. The most recent example of this is in respect of the role of the Ministry of Agriculture, Fisheries and Food (MAFF) in decisions concerning the safety of meat. Consumers distrusted a decision-making structure that seemed only to consider the interests of the industry. So complete was the breakdown in trust, that the debate on food safety was not about whether or not the status quo should prevail but what was the best alternative.

The role that government should play in our individual lives forms part of a broader political debate, and views on this will largely depend on individual philosophies. However, there has been a trend towards less government intervention in our daily lives than was once the case. Our research into consumer attitudes towards the government's role in food safety shows clearly that consumers resent limitations being placed on choice. But in direct contrast, they also expect that the government's priority should be the protection of public health and that intervention is necessary when this could be compromized. Phrases such as the 'nanny state' have tended to obscure rather than illuminate the nature of the discussion. No one seriously questions the role of the government in the analysis and control of risk. The question is better formulated as 'when should we regulate and how?'

## A place for regulation

In some situations it will be necessary for the government to intervene. When dealing with complex products, provision of information alone may not be adequate; for example, we wouldn't expect to have to decide for ourselves whether or not a new drug was safe. In some situations a product ban or withdrawal may be necessary. When dealing with broader issues, particularly ones where we are uncertain about the long-term consequences, it may be necessary for a moratorium to be introduced until the facts are better understood and further research has been conducted. A balance has to be reached.

CA has always advocated that markets should be able to operate freely and that consumers should be able to exercise choice. Our approach can be summarized as follows:

'ensuring that markets work effectively and are not constrained in ways that reduce consumer choice ... In many areas, the best way to promote consumer choice is to allow consumers to choose freely for themselves'(-Consumers' Association 1996).

However, we have also been clear to point out that the costs and benefits of regulation need to be carefully considered:

'regulation normally carries a cost, some if not all is borne by consumers. Consumers may be willing to accept this, but only if the cost is proportionate to the benefits gained in terms of health, safety, fairer trading practices and better information' (Consumers' Association 1993).

The challenge in developing a new approach to dealing with risk is to develop a mechanism for ensuring more robust and socially acceptable decisions about when and how the government should intervene. It involves determining where the balance should fall between the two fundamental consumer principles of safety and choice.

# Communicating about risk

## Uncertainty and openness

Enabling consumers to make their own decisions about the risks they are prepared to take requires that they have sufficient information and understanding to do so. There will, however, be some situations when we don't know what the risk is—too many uncertainties may remain to enable proper quantification and therefore to enable consumers to make an informed choice. But this can be incredibly difficult in the closed decision-making environment described above where uncertainties are not openly acknowledged. We may often be unaware that we have not been presented with all of the facts.

The introduction of a Freedom of Information Act should go some way to addressing these concerns, although it is still unclear what effect this will have on transparency of decision-making in practice. Information needs to be put into the public domain in an active way. As part of this there needs to be a review of exactly what is meant by 'commercially confidential'. This should not be used as an excuse to prevent disclosure of information that is in the public interest. The problem is compounded by the lack of openness about the level of scientific understanding. If there are uncertainties they should be made clear. Continuing false reassurances of safety can only prove counter-productive in the longer term.

It is clear that at the moment, the way that advice and information about health risks is provided leads to confusion and suspicion. The problem with the UK approach was summed up by the former Secretary of State for Health who, when commenting on consumer reaction to the BSE crisis, stated that we were dealing with 'mad consumers' rather than mad cows. We need to move away from this desire to defend the exclusivity of the current structures, rather than seeking to explain or respond to concerns, when judgements are challenged.

The CA focus groups conducted shortly after the publication of the White Paper on a Food Standards Agency (Ministry of Agriculture, Fisheries and Food 1998) suggested that consumers were becoming increasingly apathetic about information on food. They felt that government information was inconsistent and unclear. The balance and scale of information that was provided was felt to fluctuate and was therefore confusing. If they were given information about a potential risk, consumers also wanted this to be backed up with clear information about action they could take to reduce that risk.

Against the background of such a complex debate, there is no simple answer to the question of risk communication and how we should approach it, yet it is essential to our future security that we do just that.

## A new approach

As set out above, risk communication in its current form is predominantly one-way, and comes at the end of the risk analysis process. But risk communication must not be seen as a public relations exercise—putting the gloss on decisions that have already been made. The only way that this can be effectively achieved is by involving consumers from the beginning of the process. This will help to increase the robustness of the decisions that are made by ensuring that we are addressing the right questions from the very beginning. For example, before we start to see genetically modified animal products, we need to consider whether or not consumers will find genetic modification of animals acceptable—under any circumstances. It may be that if this leads to a reduction in the number of cases of food poisoning, e.g. by modifying animals to make them disease resistant, some consumers would find it acceptable; others may not. However, we need to ensure that we have the public debate at the right level before we are confronted with the likely rejection and then the corresponding inability to trace these developments through the food chain. As consumers are more actively involved within the decision-making process and become more familiar with the issues under discussion, they will become better informed and more able to participate. This, in turn, should improve the quality of decisions that are made.

The first stage involves establishing trust. This involves operating in an open and transparent manner and being upfront about any uncertainties that still remain. To be truly participatory, decision-making has to be transparent. It also means ensuring independence. It is important that updates are given once the initial media interest in an issue has faded. If a decision has to be made to regulate in some way to control the potential risk, this needs to be put in context to ensure that the public fully understands the reasons why the course of action was considered necessary. In the case of BSE, for example, an ongoing dialogue about the uncertainties that remained and any new scientific research that was under way would enable greater understanding of the government's reasons for deciding to take action.

Any information about risk also needs to be put in context. There have frequently been attempts to develop scales of risk, but this can often be counter-productive. It fails to acknowledge issues where there is insufficient knowledge to quantify the risk. It can also fail to acknowledge the multifactorial nature of risks that can't be shown on a simple scale. If risk communication is effective, this scale may also change as behaviour does. However, consumers do need to be given clear information about relative risks. One of the many advantages that we see with the new Food Standards Agency is that it will be a 'one stop shop' for information about food. The Agency will have a Risk Communication Unit, and this should be able to explain more immediate food safety problems in relation to the foods that we should be eating to sustain good health in the long term. If, for example, a survey should indicate a safety problem, the results need to be backed up by information that puts them into context, explaining their significance.

The media through which this information is provided will also be key to its success—the information needs to reach the desired audience. It also needs to be communicated in a language that is readily understandable and relevant to people's own experiences. Involving relevant stakeholders will be crucial for ensuring that it is consistently and effectively communicated in a way that is meaningful. This should also help to ensure that any dissenting views about the appropriate course of action can be addressed openly. Involving 'on the ground' professionals will also help to ensure the dissemination of information. The CA survey looking at trust in information about food found that health professionals were considered to be most trustworthy. These professionals, however, are often reliant on the government for the information and advice they provide. Perceived independence is clearly an important factor, as has been demonstrated by other survey findings (Marris and Langford 1996; European Commission 1997). As pointed out in Chapter 3, friends and family have been shown to be a reliable source of information. Independence of government and commercial biases is seen as important and therefore consumer and environmental groups rank highly. Doctors and scientists are also considered to be quite trustworthy.

Ways also need to be considered to ensure that information is kept in the public mind, once it has ceased to be a major news story. Advice needs to be reiterated and information updated (*Which?* 1997). It is also important to remember that risk communication doesn't always have to be negative—it can also have a positive message about how to improve the quality of life. As other contributors argue, risk communication has to be seen as an ongoing dialogue, not just an add-on at the end of the risk analysis process. It is not just a case of making consumers understand, but is about improving the quality of the debate. Though we need to get better at explaining some scientific points—notably the difference between absolute and relative risk— the answer is not simply to 'educate' consumers until they understand the science—this assumes that the process remains solely within the scientific template. Merely being more open about the uncertainties we face, while helpful, underestimates the task in hand. The key issue is trust.

## Effectively involving consumers

It is now widely recognized that the first step towards improving the quality of the risk debate is ensuring greater public participation in the regulatory process (Health and Safety Executive 1999). How to achieve this and measure whether or not we have been successful is more complex. However, there is no doubt that the time has now come to move on from the intellectual discussions and to actually start to put some of the theory into practice. The government needs to experiment actively with methods of public participation. It is only by openly debating future developments and attempting to reach consensus on the level of risk that we can start to make acceptable provision for uncertainties.

This needs to take place at several levels. Consumer representatives need to be appointed to key decision-making bodies, particularly expert advisory committees. Although this is now starting to happen in the UK, there has been little progress at European and international level. But public involvement needs to start even before this—when the problem is defined and decisions are made about the scope of the risk assessment. Others steps need to be taken, for example, holding meetings in public and inviting observers to attend. More generally, research needs to be undertaken to enable policy-makers to have a greater understanding of consumer attitudes that can feed into policy decisions.

Methods of ensuring greater public involvement in decision-making have already been tried in some situations—usually at a local level. The problem is that they have rarely been used to increase public involvement in national government, or more globally. Several mechanisms are now available, many of which have been tried more widely in the US, Germany, and the Netherlands. They include the use of referenda, deliberative polling (a representative group of people are invited to listen to a short debate on an issue before voting on it), citizens' juries (as described in the following chapter, a representative group of people hearing evidence on an issue before reaching a verdict), citizens' workshops (a lower scale version citizens' juries), consensus conferences (larger versions of citizens' juries), and Internet forums. So far there has been little work done on assessing the relative merits of these mechanisms. Some will be both time consuming and costly. Some may be better suited to dealing with specific issues, others such as consensus conferences, may be more appropriate when debating issues of uncertainty. Consideration needs to be given to what is most appropriate under the circumstances: it may be most effective to use a combination of methods (Consumers' Association 1998).

We are used to taking a purely scientific approach to deliberations about risk, and therefore it is easy to dismiss such methods until there is conclusive evidence of their effectiveness. However, consumer participation isn't necessarily going to have an obvious, measurable result. There are no wrong and right answers. The results may differ from government policy, and even surprise other interested groups, but that is not to say that it has not been effective.

In summary, what we are arguing is that the structure, participants, and process are the key to creating the environment where a more positive dialogue can take place. Ultimately controlling risk is about controlling our futures—and reaching agreement on the most socially acceptable way this can be achieved.

# REFERENCES

Advisory Committee on Novel Foods and Processes (1995). *Annual Report*. Advisory Committee on Novel Foods and Processes, London.

Consumers' Association (1993). *Response to the Department of Trade and Industry's (DTI) consultation on deregulation*. Consumers' Association, London.

Consumers' Association (1996). *Making markets work*. Consumers' Association, London.

Consumers' Association (1997). *Gene cuisine—a consumer agenda for genetically modified foods*, (S. Davies), policy report. Consumers' Association, London.

Consumers' Association (1998). *Consumer representation*, (S. Dee), policy report. Consumers' Association, London.

Consumers' Association (1999). *Confronting Risk—a new approach to food safety* (S. Davies) policy report. Consumers' Association, London.

Consumers' Association, Sainsbury's, and Unilever (1998). *Confronting risk—finding new approaches to risk*, report of a roundtable held on 10 October 1997, Royal College of Surgeons, London.

Davies, S. and Todd, S. (1996). An independent food agency. *Consumer Policy Review*, **6** (3), 82–6.

European Commission (1997). *Europeans and modern biotechnology*, Eurobarometer Survey 46.1. DGVII of the Commission, Brussels.

Health and Safety Executive (1999). *Risk assessment and risk management*. Inter-departmental Liaison Group on Risk Assessment, Health and Safety Executive, London.

Marris, C. and Langford, I. (1996). No cause for alarm. *New Scientist*, 28 September, pp. 36–9.

Ministry of Agriculture, Fisheries and Food (1998). *The Food Standards Agency—a force for change*. Ministry of Agriculture, Fisheries and Food, London.

MORI (1999). *Public attitudes to risk*. MORI, London.

Scientific Committee for Animal Nutrition (SCAN) (1996). *Report on the safety for animals of certain genetically modified maize lines notified by Ciba-Geigy in accordance with Directive 90/220 for feedingstuff use* (opinion expressed on 13 December 1996). Scientific Committee for Animal Nutrition, London.

Scientific Committee for Food (SCF) (1996). *Opinion on the potential for adverse health effects from the consumption of genetically modified maize* (13 December 1996). Scientific Committee for Food, London.

Sheppard, J. (1998). Risky business. *Consumer Policy Review*, **8** (2), 58–62.

Stern, P. C. and Fineberg, H. V. (ed.) (1996). *Understanding risk: informing decisions in a democratic society*. National Research Council, London.

*Which?* (1997). *Is our health in crisis? Which*, September, pp. 22–5. Consumers' Association, London.

# 14 Negotiating risks to public health—models for participation

Anna Coote, *the King's Fund, London* and
Jane Franklin, *South Bank University, London*

## Introduction

Risks to public health are infinitely varied. Some take the form of a catastrophe threatening the lives of complete local populations, such as a volcanic eruption or a chemical emission. Some constitute serious and widespread risks to health, such as infected meat, polluted water, extremes of heat or cold, or a major 'flu epidemic. And some arise from individual lifestyles, such as sporting accidents, or the consequences of eating too much fat or sugar. These categories are not discrete or fixed. They can overlap and merge, they can mutate, reproduce, and diverge. Yet for as long as public health remains a concern of public policy, risks must somehow be addressed and strategies must be devised for dealing with them.

Some risks to public health, such as new variant CJD, are more difficult than others to predict or assess. As illustrated all too clearly in earlier chapters, they tend to undermine relationships of trust between politicians, experts, and the public, and challenge conventional approaches to policy- and decision-making. Initially, this poses a problem for policy-makers, but we argue that, in the longer term, it opens the way for a different approach that fits more closely with the changing nature of risk and with a more mature, open, and accountable polity.

This chapter offers, firstly, a perspective on some of the key problems. Secondly, it sets out the need for a new political dialogue as a key element in tackling these problems. Finally, it considers the key features of *citizens' juries* and their usefulness in promoting such dialogue, and reports on some practical experiences.

# The key challenges

## The changing nature of risk

Ulrich Beck and Anthony Giddens have argued that as modern society matures, we are confronted more and more with the consequences of the many decisions and choices that have been made in the interest of industrial and social development (Beck 1998; Giddens 1998). Risks associated with BSE, salmonella from eggs, and antibiotic-resistant bacteria are characteristic of social change and reflect the impact of human intervention in natural processes. With these risks, we become aware of what we have done to the world we live in. The policy problem arises when decisions have to be made about how to deal with these risks and how to communicate them to the public. Scientists often disagree: science indeed is often the culprit. People look to doctors and politicians to advise them on how to deal with health risks that could not be, and indeed were not, predicted.

The unpredictability of these risks is enough to challenge current policy processes, which rely on the possibility of prediction and assessment, so that decisions can be made which will make the risk environment safe. For example, evidence that BSE could be passed on to humans in the form of CJD was largely circumstantial and difficult for experts to assess. When news of a possible link hit the headlines, 'action was forced on a reluctant government by a concerned public' (Tindale 1998). Government action and advice was reactive and piecemeal, and in the ensuring confusion, individuals were left to balance the odds for themselves. Some stopped eating beef altogether, others took a fatalistic approach and decided to 'risk it'. Subsequent policy decisions, such as the banning of beef on the bone, confused and irritated the public rather than reassuring them—not the basis of responsible and effective public health policy.

What kind of policy would enable effective decision-making in the context of unpredictable risks? At present, the government works within a policy framework that links and balances individual responsibility for health with the duty of the state to provide health care (DoH 1998). Within this framework, the ideal is that information on health and health risks is accurate, understandable, and credible and that, in the light of this information, people can either make decisions and take responsibility for their own and their family's health, or accept with confidence the government's decision to take action on their behalf. This can *only* work with risks that can be assessed, predicted, and known, e.g. the risk of sexually transmitted diseases, teenage pregnancy, coronary heart disease, lung cancer. However, with the new risks we have described, the links between information and responsibility become more problematic in principle (rather than only in practice).

How can individuals make decisions about their own and their family's health if there *is no* precise and accurate information about risks? How can governments inform and reassure individuals about risks that are unknowable, unpredictable, and about which experts disagree? At this stage it becomes evident that risk is political—demanding a new kind of political engagement between experts, politicians, and the public in which trust is pivotal.

## Trust revisited

The need to manage risks to public health effectively and the need to generate trust in political relationships coincide and are dependent on each other. In dealing with health risks, people have to make judgements which depend on how they perceive their future life chances. This depends, in turn, on how they view the information they receive and the integrity of its sources. If they do not trust those sources, how are they to make judgements with any confidence? Yet the capacity of experts and politicians to inspire trust is itself shaped by the nature of risk. If outcomes are unpredictable, they cannot act or advise with any certainty. Consequently, each new public health crisis tends to put a new strain on the government's credibility. Trust itself is in danger of spiralling into decline.

Trust was never very strong between people and politicians, but it is decomposing in new ways. The reasons are many and complex—and not all are directly attributable to the changing nature of risk. Overall, the decline of trust has to do with illusion and disillusion. So many things in politics are not what they seem. For example, politicians can now speak, for the first time in history, directly to millions of people. They can communicate across vast distances—providing an illusion of proximity thanks to new technologies and the mass media. Yet the actual distances between the electorate and their elected representatives can be very great. And these are keenly felt, both in a horizontal sense—geographical distance from central government—and in a vertical sense, where multiple layers of decision-making are reinforced by a culture of secrecy and by informal and largely hidden social networks and alliances, through which information and consent must be filtered.

In order to communicate with vast numbers across vast distances, politicians play by the rules of the mass media. Accordingly, the complex issues and arguments that lie behind most policy decisions are considered unpalatable for mass audiences. Political leaders must strive instead to be media heroes to win the hearts of the voter. The projection of personality, the careful choice of clothing, or 'human interest' details and anecdotes—all these are used to convey impressions and stimulate feelings. An illusion is created as the appearance of personal candour and the 'human touch' become proxies for political honesty and trustworthiness. In a contrary twist to the feminist maxim that the 'personal is political', the political is reduced to the personal. The effect is to generate suspicion rather than under-standing.

## Mutual distrust

Indeed, there is low trust on both sides. A widely held view among politicians is that ordinary members of the public are incapable of grasping complex issues or forming views of any relevance. They assume they will believe anything they read in the newspapers, that their opinions are shaped by narrow and selfish concerns, that they are generally apathetic and will not take time or trouble to consider anything which does not affect them directly. It follows that, if people are gullible, selfish, and irresponsible, it would be futile or dangerous to involve them in any kind of dialogue or decision-making.

At the same time, there is a widely held view among the public that the whole process of decision-making is hopelessly impermeable and that whatever they do or say will make no difference. Many people believe that, even if they were to make a contribution, it would be worthless—a fear fuelled by the fact that they have never tried to participate and therefore feel inexperienced and unqualified. The only option left, it seems, is to vest responsibility in politicians and other experts who put themselves forward for the job, even though they intuitively fear their failings and suspect their integrity. This mutual distrust has the effect of undermining the people's democratic practice, justifying their continued exclusion from decision-making, and shoring up a moribund relationship between people and politicians.

Can we recover? What can be done to create the foundations for a mature, high-trust democracy in which information and decisions about risks can be shared? When personal relationships break down, they can sometimes be mended by careful consideration and respectful dialogue between the parties involved. Could something similar help to rebuild political relationships?

# Toward a new political dialogue

## From risk communication to negotiation

Current debates about communicating risks to public health are beginning to explore such possibilities. The Department of Health (1997; Chapter 1) has recognized that policy-making around the issue of risk has evolved:

'*from* an original emphasis on public misperceptions of risk, which tended to treat all deviations from expert estimates as products of ignorance or stupidity, *via* empirical investigation of what actually does cause concern and why, *to* approaches which promote risk communication as a two-way process in which both 'expert' and 'lay' perspectives should inform each other'.

Viewed in this light, risk communication strategies can facilitate a dialogue between experts and the public—a two-way sharing of information that moves the debate into the public domain and promises to open up decision-making processes to scrutiny (Chapter 15). The overall objective is to find more effective ways of securing the public health against risk, and to establish a safe environment and an element of trust between expert and public opinion. However, this approach still rests on the assumption that risks can be calculated and predicted. If, as we have suggested, this is no longer the case with some risks, we are entering territory where decisions are required, but where there may be no right or wrong answer. This implies a need to *negotiate*, rather than merely *communicate* risks.

While 'communication' implies (or should imply) a two-way conversation for sharing information and perspectives, 'negotiation' can be seen as a multiple engagement of diverse forms of knowledge and experience. Negotiation is not a conversation that begins and ends, but one that continues, where the ambiguities and uncertainties can be laid out and confronted. It accepts that both expert and lay knowledge may be insufficient or irrelevant—not up to the job of assessing or avoiding risks. It aims to accommodate, rather than overcome that insufficiency and reconcile all parties to the fallibilities of the others. It is not about finding better ways of re-establishing reassurance and safety, but of dealing with uncertainty in a strong political environment, where trust is generated through open dialogue. It works to build political relationships that can tolerate conflicting views and difference of opinion, so that politicians and experts can say what they do and do not know, while individuals and groups can question and legitimately contest and contribute to political decisions. The success of such a strategy requires mature political relations, a commitment to planning for uncertainty and appropriate mechanisms for public involvement in decision-making. We discuss each of these briefly in turn.

## Mature political relations

As things stand we, the public, look to politicians to advise us on how to deal with risks. We expect clear answers, viable solutions, consistency, and certainty. We cannot tolerate it when politicians fail to deliver—yet we know, instinctively, that they often cannot succeed. The media on our behalf—and in our name—persecutes politicians and experts who fail to provide a clear answer, or change their minds, or disagree with their colleagues. This is not unlike a dysfunctional relationship between adolescents and their parents. We still want our politician-parents to be infallible. Yet we strongly suspect they are not and consequently despise them. For their part, the politicians dissemble and deceive, scared of triggering mood swings, sulks, withdrawal of love and affection. They do not trust their voter-children to produce a mature response (Coote 1998).

The implications of 'risk society' (Beck 1992; Giddens 1994) for the conduct of public policy-making is that we must grow up and develop an adult-to-adult relationship with our politicians, as well as with 'experts'. An adult-to-adult relationship does not imply that everyone knows the same as everyone else, but that we all know something, that no one is omniscient. Ideally, we respect each other's knowledge and experience—we are not over-awed or diminished by any of it, nor are we slighting or disdainful. We interact and are interdependent, as human beings who are different but equal.

We need a new political culture which supports an informed and reasonable scepticism about scientific and 'expert' knowledge. Not Luddite rejection or slavish acquiescence, but somewhere between. That requires clarity and transparency about the interests of experts—professional or commercial. It requires as much public access as possible to their knowledge and their deliberations, and wide public debate about what they say: their ideas, their evidence, and their interpretations.

More important still, we need a new political culture that enables politicians to admit they do not have the answer to every question, that enables them to admit they may be wrong, and that applauds rather than ridicules them when they own up to ignorance or change their minds. The politicians must learn to act as 'honest broker' between the public and the experts. That means letting the public in on the secrets of the experts, including the well-guarded 'secret' of their fallibility. It means letting the public in on the limits of the politicians' own knowledge and power. It also means identifying and publicizing the different interests involved in decisions, making it possible to negotiate openly between them. That the public has an interest both as citizens/taxpayers and as users of goods and services, should be well understood.

## Planning for uncertainty

A successful strategy for negotiating risk requires an appreciation of the scope and limitations of politics and government. Mainstream political parties no longer envisage an ideal end-state to which they aspire. Neither science nor economics can be relied upon to provide certain predictions. The further we push out the boundaries of human knowledge, the more we manufacture new uncertainties and the more we should know how impossible it is to be certain about anything. Therefore, government must commit itself to planning for uncertainty as one of its major functions.

Planning for uncertainty requires a clear sense of the principles that guide policy-making: we may not know the shape of things to come or where we want to end up, but we can form a view about *why* and *how* we are travelling. Planning for uncertainty calls for negotiation rather than communication. It demands clarity and openness about what we do know—a realistic appraisal of the evidence at our disposal, and a deep understanding of the present (not marred by a rose-tinted view of the past). It involves knowing that we cannot travel backwards to old certainties. And it requires laws and institutions that safeguard and promote the guiding principles, that are consistent with the evidence, and that allow for devolved and flexible decision-making in the future: enabling where possible, prescribing only when necessary.

## Appropriate mechanisms for public involvement

If mature political relations and a commitment to planning for uncertainty are prerequisites of a strategy for negotiating risk, a question that remains is how to develop appropriate mechanisms for negotiation. In particular, what are the most effective ways of involving the public? A range of options is already available for bringing the views of the public into a decision-making process. Well established models include opinion polls and surveys, focus groups and public meetings; innovations include citizens' panels and forums, deliberative polls, and citizens' juries. Old ones can be adapted and new ones developed. An effective approach will have to meet certain criteria. For example, the negotiation of risk is about multiple layers of decision-making, which means including the voices of all the relevant stakeholders. Dialogue and discussion take place in an arena of conflicting and sometimes antagonistic opinions and interests, and will need careful facilitation. The process of decision-making has to be flexible and able to accommodate an outcome where there is no consensus about a 'right' or 'wrong' answer.

# A practical form of engagement

Work carried out by the Institute for Public Policy Research (IPPR) between 1993 and 1998 offers some useful insights. The Institute conducted a series of pilot citizens' juries and subsequently developed a Public Involvement

Programme to facilitate the exchange of ideas and skills between organizations engaged in innovation in this area.

The experiment with citizens' juries grew out of a critique of conventional approaches to public involvement. These were seen to have various shortcomings. For example, a typical 'communications strategy' would all too often treat the public as passive recipients of information or opinion provided by experts—notwithstanding recent recognition of the need for dialogue. A 'consultation exercise' would often bypass important stake-holders and leave no room for genuine debate. A public meeting would provide a theatre for the rehearsal of fixed positions. An opinion survey would seek the views of the public but fail to provide any relevant information. A focus group would leave participants in the dark about how their contribution would be used in the future. And so on.

## What are citizens' juries?

The citizens' jury, adapted for the UK from models pioneered in Germany and the US, appeared to overcome some of these problems. Briefly, a group is convened of between 12 and 16 ordinary citizens who are intended approximately to match the profile of the local community. The jurors sit for up to four days and are asked to address one or more specific questions. They are given extensive background information in the form of written and oral evidence. They cross-examine a range of 'witnesses' and can call for additional evidence. They discuss the issue in depth, in small groups and in moderated plenary sessions. They are not required to reach a verdict (unanimous or majority); their conclusions are recorded and presented to the commissioning authority only after the jurors themselves have approved the report.

## Some practical experiences

IPPR, working with Opinion Leader Research—a commercial company which carried out the recruitment and moderation—has organized more than a dozen citizens' juries (including the original pilot series) for a range of organizations—among them health authorities, local authorities, a regulatory body, and a large voluntary organization. The juries addressed a variety of policy issues ranging from healthcare priorities and planning local amenities, to tackling local unemployment, regulating television for 'taste and decency', and improving services for people with mental illness living in the community. The experience has been documented and analysed elsewhere (Coote and Lenaghan 1997; Delap 1998). We do not claim that citizens' juries are an ideal model. However, the practical and theoretical work carried out by IPPR and associated organizations has helped to demonstrate how the key features of this approach can affect the politics as well as the process of public involvement. In summary, these features are concerned with the selection of participants, the deployment of time and information, the opportunity for scrutiny and deliberation, collective decision-making, independence, and openness.

Jurors are recruited using social research techniques to provide a broadly (though not scientifically) representative sample of the local population. There is, of course, an element of self-selection, since individuals must agree to participate. But jurors are not experienced activists or civic leaders, and people are drawn in who would not normally choose to take part in any political process. The amount of time set aside for discussion and the importance attached to informing the participants marks this model out from most others—and the effect is intensified because only small numbers are involved.

Participants are given a chance to cross-examine witnesses and discuss the matter at length, both with witnesses and among themselves. This means that they are better able to apply the information and consider the question, and that the process is informed by lay as well as by expert opinion. Skilled moderators are there to ensure that the discussions are open and fair, and not dominated by a few forceful personalities. Jurors forge their conclusions in a group. They are not forced to agree: individual opinions are surveyed at the beginning and end of the session; these and any minority views are recorded in the jurors' final report. Nevertheless, the jury model encourages consensus building.

A citizens' jury is intended to be independent of the commissioning organization. The jurors themselves have a degree of control over their agenda and how they consider the question before them. They 'own' their conclusions, in that they must approve the report of the jury before it is submitted to the commissioning body. The sessions are open to observers, including media representatives, and the report is in the public domain. The commissioning organization is expected to make public the fact that the jury has been convened and the question put to it, to publicize the jury's findings, to respond within a set time, and either to follow the jurors' recommendations or to explain publicly why not.

## Strengths and weaknesses as a risk negotiation mechanism

There are, inevitably, weaknesses in the jury model. It involves very small numbers of people. It is not scientifically representative. It does not give voice to specific interest groups (although in practice the jury organizers usually convene an advisory group to help frame the question and design the agenda to make sure that local stakeholders are involved). It cannot cope with a range of different languages. It costs around £30 000 or more for a four-day jury, which puts it beyond the reach of many organizations. And the fact that it is generally a one-off exercise, with jurors disbanded after the session is over, means that it cannot address policy issues as they develop over time.

However, what matters for this discussion is how the key features of the jury model can contribute constructively to the negotiation of risk. The manner of recruitment reaches parts of the population other models do not touch. The opportunity for scrutiny and deliberation, when combined in a generous time frame with plentiful background information, makes it possible for participants to consider complex issues in depth and detail. The building of consensus through informed and extended deliberation is a hallmark of effective negotiation. The independence of the process affects the status of the participants: they become subjects in a policy debate, rather than objects of a research or public relations exercise. And openness lends credibility to their findings.

Practical experience with this approach to public involvement has demonstrated that members of the public, once invited, are very willing to take part and thoroughly enjoy themselves. They quickly become competent and confident decision-makers, and are able to address complex issues and questions. They are swift to detect bias or special pleading on the part of witnesses, and they are ready to accept the practical constraints within which policy decisions have to be taken. They readily adopt a community perspective, thinking on behalf of others, not just themselves—and often change their minds during the process. In short, they defy the assumptions that politicians and 'experts' routinely make about the public. All these factors help to generate trust on both sides. However, for trust to be sustained on the public side, it is vital that the jurors' efforts are seen to be taken seriously enough to make an impact on policy and practice.

The features we have described can be combined in different ways in different models to achieve different effects. Their usefulness will depend on how far they are appropriate to the task in hand. What is the issue for negotiation? Who is initiating the process? What is at stake? What are the practical constraints of time and cost? In what capacity is the public invited to participate? (The public has complex identities and different interests which may conflict—for example, as service users or consumers, as members of special interest groups, as employees, neighbours and community members, voters and taxpayers.) Some mechanisms will work better than others in differing circumstances. The important thing is to match purpose to method, always pushing at the boundaries to improve opportunities to inform and empower the public, accommodate change, build mutual confidence, and make better decisions.

# Conclusions

If policy makers are inventive and can think creatively they should be able to adapt to the changing nature of risks to public health. Individuals are now making significant choices in the context of conflicting information amid a growing scepticism as to the competence of experts—increasingly taking it upon themselves to make decisions about their own bodies and their own health. For their part, institutions—political and scientific—might recognize their role in the manufacture of risk and their capacity to change, adapt, and invent new strategies to cope with the more complex decision-making processes demanded by those risks. The capacity to change is all-important. As Ulrich Beck says, we must all 'be prepared to jump over [our] own shadows'(Beck 1997). Politicians may find to their advantage that it is possible to spread responsibility for decision-making. There could be less pressure on them to give infallible advice to the public and less pressure on scientists to provide absolute proof.

We have argued that in public health policy a complex strategy of risk negotiation may often be more appropriate than the simple communication of risks to the public, or even two-way communication. The strategy must itself be open and flexible, giving space to uncertainty and unpredictability, and enabling creative and democratic thinking to work alongside traditional mechanisms of decision-making. Its implementation need not be dramatic, but it would represent a radical adjustment to social change, driven by the imperative of the risks themselves, which refuse to be dealt with in traditional ways. It would shift the focus of policy-making, from a combination of paternalism and individual risk management, to risk politics in which trust is generated to provide a sound basis for democratic consent.

## REFERENCES

Beck, U. (1992). *Risk society: towards a new modernity*. Sage, London.

Beck, U. (1997). *The Reinvention of Politics*, Polity Press, Cambridge.

Beck, U. (1998). Politics of risk society. In *The politics of risk society*, (ed. J. Franklin). Polity Press, Cambridge.

Coote, A. and Lenaghan, J. (1997). *Citizens' juries: theory into practice*. Institute for Public Policy Research, London.

Coote, A. (1998*a*). Risk and public policy: towards a high trust democracy. In *The politics of risk society*, (ed. J. Franklin). Polity Press, Cambridge.

Delap, C. (1998). *Making better decisions*. Institute for Public Policy Research, London.

Department of Health (1997). *Communicating about risks to public health: pointers to good practice*. Department of Health, London. (Second edition 1998, The Stationery Office)

Department of Health (1998). *Our healthier nation,* Green Paper. HMSO, London.

Giddens, A. (1994). *Beyond left and right: the future of radical politics*. Polity Press, Cambridge.

Giddens, A. (1998). Risk society: the context of British politics. In *The politics of risk society*, (ed. J. Franklin). Polity Press, Cambridge.

Tindale, S. (1998). Procrastination, precaution and the global gamble. In *The politics of risk society*, (ed. J. Franklin). Polity Press, Cambridge.

# 15 The identification and management of risk: opening up the process

David Coles
*Department of Health*

## Introduction

In recent years there have been important developments in the government's approach to risk communication. It might once have been possible to take a 'government knows best' approach, simply informing the public that a risk has been identified, telling people not to worry, and stating what the government intends to do about it. As will be abundantly clear from previous chapters, this is no longer acceptable or appropriate in a modern information-based society. This much is common ground in debates about risk communication. It is recognized that there has been a significant loss of public confidence in the government's ability to handle risk and to protect public health. Regaining trust requires much greater transparency of the risk assessment and risk management processes and more public involvement in decisions. Given the key role played by the independent scientific committees set up to advise government, a good deal of the risk communication debate has focused on demands to 'open up' this part of the system. At the same time, the debate has highlighted other issues to do with the relationship between advice and policy decisions. This chapter outlines some of these issues, and then discusses how governments both in the UK and overseas—particularly in Australia and New Zealand—are responding to calls for greater openness in their regulatory processes.

## Advice and policy: some issues

To develop policy on public health issues, government regulators need scientific information in order to make an assessment of the hazard and the extent of any consequent risk to public health. As set out in the Preface to Part III, departments make use of a network of expert advisory committees and associated working groups, particularly when advice is needed on complex or controversial risks. The aim is to obtain independent, authoritative advice. (Other sources include the Office of Science and Technology and the Chief Scientific Advisor, research councils, research committees, industry, various interest groups, individual experts, workshops, and a range of Non-Departmental Public Bodies and *ad hoc* groups.) Despite the increasing demands for the public to be represented in the process of advising government, examination of the system has not only been prompted by external criticism. Recent episodes have encouraged considerable discussion across government and among the committees themselves. Linked with issues of transparency and openness are fundamental questions about the proper relationship between scientific advice and policy.

Any supposition that policy can be based on science *alone* can place committees, as well as government, in a very difficult position. Government may be accused of ignoring risks and giving in to pressure from industry or other lobby groups or conversely of acting like a 'nanny state' in cases where the public feels well able to make its own decisions. Such criticisms may be unjust, but they will not be dispelled by insisting that policy is effectively *dictated by* scientific advice. In the first place, shifts in public attitudes have led to much less willingness to leave problem-solving to the experts. Perhaps more importantly, people can perfectly well see that policy involves value judgements as well as science. To pretend otherwise merely causes the credibility of the committees to suffer as well. Indeed, presenting advisory committees as being responsible for policy can increase suspicion that they are failing to take contrary views into account or even colluding with government in some cover-up of the truth. The end result is to damage public confidence not only in government, but in the whole risk assessment and management process.

Recognizing the above points leaves open the key question of whether advisory committees should simply carry out an *assessment* of the science or also address issues of risk *management*. Some scientists argue that their role should lie purely with risk assessments based on scientific evidence alone. Other factors—such as value judgements or public perceptions—should be considered by others, as part of a *separate* risk management process. However, in reality the science is rarely clear-cut and there is frequently a lot of uncertainty associated with the evidence, particularly where public health issues are concerned. Consequently, it may not be possible to separate 'pure science' from value judgements. As a result, conclusions often cannot be based solely on factual scientific data but must rely on the experience and expertise of individual committee members. However, the danger is that there may be no explicit recognition of which value judgements are being incorporated, and when.

This situation has been a cause for concern, and different committees have responded in different ways (which in itself can make the committee system's role seem ambiguous). Some are wary of being expected to go into the realms of advice on risk management strategies or even on policy. They see these as requiring judgements that may lie beyond their areas of expertise. Other committees have felt that their particular remit may call for provision of advice on risk management, and have therefore sought to bring a wider range of expertise and experience into the committee. Chapter 11 describes how one such committee, the Advisory Committee on Novel Food Products (ACNFP), has set about this process; another example is the Gene Therapy Advisory Committee (GTAC).

Moving on to the issue of openness, many committees have historically been constituted to provide advice to ministers—often through their departmental secretariat—rather than to the outside world. Because of this, some have in the past effectively worked behind closed doors. One result is that there may be little or no awareness of their role—or even their existence—outside their specialist working circle. This can cause problems for the committees themselves. For example, unorthodox views from outside individuals may get a wide airing in the media without any reference back to the relevant committees—or any acknowledgement that they may well have already taken account of any evidence supporting these contrary views. It also means that there is very little understanding by the public—and indeed by many professionals—of the committees' important role in the protection of health and the challenges of fulfilling it. From the committees' point of view, this can contribute to both politicians and the public having unrealistic expectations of them, wanting black and white answers to risk issues and demanding a 'no-risk' environment.

Even if such pitfalls are avoided, the process of using scientific advice can present both ministers and committees with difficult problems, especially on issues of particular sensitivity or public concern. For example, suppose a committee is charged to produce a risk assessment based solely on the scientific evidence. Once this has been completed, a considered policy cannot be produced until other relevant factors are taken into account. (These may include the views of the general public or particular stakeholders, or input from others with social, psychological, financial, or regulatory expertise.) But this need presents a dilemma. If the scientific assessment is published straight away, politicians may be put under enormous pressure to come up with 'instant answers' on how to deal with the problem. But if the committee's findings are not disclosed until an effective risk management policy has been developed, government lays itself open to accusations of non-disclosure or cover-up—and to the danger of being 'bounced' into less considered action by leaks. Clearly the ideal is for committee conclusions to be released as soon as possible. However, for this to be effective the general public—and in particular the media—must develop a more mature understanding of the *processes* involved in developing policies to protect public health. In particular, they will need to appreciate that a more transparent process will often reveal 'work in progress' contributing to risk management, rather than definitive policy conclusions. One can then begin to distinguish the processes of risk assessment, risk management, and policy development, so allowing greater opportunities for two-way communication at all stages. This should in the end lead to better and more acceptable risk management strategies.

# Current developments in the UK

Various responses to these issues are already in train. Concerns over the limitations of scientific advice and its application—as evidenced in particular by the BSE crisis—led the House of Commons Science and Technology Committee to set up an inquiry into the scientific advisory system. Currently in progress, this is looking at how government uses scientific advice, the quality of that advice, how it is organized, and how best to establish public confidence.

Meanwhile the Office of Science and Technology has already issued guidelines on the use of scientific advice (Office of Science and Technology 1997). These set out some important principles, one being that:

> 'there should be a presumption towards openness in explaining the scientific advice and its interpretation. Departments should aim to make public all the scientific evidence and analysis underlying the policy decisions on the sensitive areas covered by the guidelines. The scientific process thrives on openness, which stimulates greater critical discussion of the scientific basis of policy proposals and raises any conflicting evidence which may have been overlooked'.

Another factor driving this approach towards greater openness has been a rapidly growing awareness of the importance of communication within the risk assessment process, not simply as a means of disseminating information but as a two-way process of information exchange and input into decision-making. Consequently there has been much recent activity across a range of government departments to develop best practice. The Department of Health's programme is outlined in Chapters 16 and 20. Risk communication has also become an increasingly important topic for the Interdepartmental Liaison Group on Risk Assessment (ILGRA) which recently commissioned a benchmarking study of government practice. Some results were described in Chapter 9, and underpin a guidance document (Interdepartmental Liaison Group on Risk Assessment 1998) on how risk communication should be incorporated into the Departments' risk analysis procedures. ILGRA has also set up a subgroup to contribute to the development of risk communication across government.

A clear message emerging both in the UK and internationally is that risk communication is not just an add-on to risk assessment but needs to inform thinking through the whole process. It is recognized that this may require a 'culture shift' to take much greater account of openness, public perception and participation, and ethical issues at an early stage, and to iterate these considerations back into the assessment and management processes.

Though there is clearly a growing awareness of the need for greater transparency in the development of regulatory policy on risk, a number of issues will need to be addressed. One particularly difficult question to resolve is that of balancing openness with confidentiality, particularly in respect of material and data that is supplied 'commercial in confidence' or involves prepublication scientific research. Advisory committees often rely on good-will from researchers, based on an assumption of confidentiality, in order to gain early access to data. If this data were fully open to public scrutiny as soon as being made available to the committee, researchers would be reluctant to release relevant information until they were in a position to formally publish their results. Similar difficulties arise on other occasions when sensitive data is provided on a voluntary basis. For example, committees may receive requests for advice from a manufacturer regarding a product or process still under development.

Nevertheless, committees associated with a number of government departments are already moving towards publishing key documents related to their work. Many of the those used by both the Department of Health (DH) and MAFF, for example, have taken significant initiatives to improve openness. Some have begun to provide access to their agendas or to minutes of meetings or summaries of discussions. Others provide regular bulletins of their activities and findings to interested groups through publications such as the *Chief Medical Officer's Update* or MAFF's *Food Bulletin*. Most now also publish annual reports and registers of members' interests. The Internet is proving to be a particularly useful tool in increasing openness, as it provides quick and easy access to information. While the 'paper' circulation of publications may be very small, their content can be very widely accessed if published on the World Wide Web. Many committees are now developing and using their own web pages to disseminate information about their work. The Internet does of course open up the committee's work to an international audience. While this has the advantage of disseminating information much more widely, it may also generate much greater and more widespread demands for yet more information. In fact, openness can be very resource-intensive.

In an attempt to improve openness and also to add another dimension to their considerations, many committees now include lay, public interest, or particular interest representatives within the committee membership. As described in Chapter 11, they are finding that these can help to set committee advice in a broader context and establish a better foundation for communicating to a wider audience. Significantly, these moves are not confined to committees with a wider 'risk management' remit such as ACNFP or GTAC (see above), but also encompass some committees basing their advice solely on scientific evidence, such as the Committee on Toxicology (COT).

Other attempts to take better account of public and stakeholder values have used a variety of consultation processes including consultation papers, workshops, and open meetings. Although these have been of some use, participants are frequently self-selecting and therefore not representative of the public at large. Attention has therefore been turning recently to a broader range of public participation models, some of which are or have been used in other settings or by foreign regulators and governments.


# Models of public participation—examples from other countries

In seeking to compare experiences on public policy issues, countries such as Australia and New Zealand provide fertile ground, not least because their overall political systems and culture have traditionally had much in common with our own. In fact, both have in recent years followed a rather different and more open approach to risk regulation than the UK. For example, whereas many UK regulators are based in government departments and their expert committees are constituted to report to ministers, all regulatory bodies in Australia are independent and make their advice public without reference to ministers. In addition, Australia does not use a system of standing expert advisory committees but may set up committees on an *ad hoc* basis to address specific issues. However, New Zealand retains an expert committee structure similar to that of the UK. One specific problem for both countries lies in only having a small pool of indigenous expertise. This means that their experts are usually in high demand and can only commit themselves to a small amount of unpaid advisory work. Consequently their assessment process is slow compared to that in the UK.

In order to address the problem of limited numbers of experts and also to respond to demand for greater openness, both Australia and New Zealand have made considerable use of public consultation and participation in the decision-making process. New Zealand has also recently carried out a major review of its expert advisory committees (Smith 1997), one recommendation being that they should incorporate more lay representation.

New Zealand in particular has been at the forefront in using public consultation, possibly to the point where there is now a degree of public cynicism about the role of consultation and regulators feel a need to keep the public continually informed of the extent to which the government takes their views into account. There is a statutory obligation to consult on any new public health policy—although there are often problems identifying exactly what constitutes new policy. As a result it normally takes at least a year to develop a policy paper, with every submission arising from a consultation having to be carefully read and annotated and the original proposals redrafted to take account of them. Of course not every submission received has to be incorporated into the revised draft but, as all are recoverable under New Zealand's Freedom of Information Act, considered reasons have to be given for not including them. Consequently the consultation process is both time-consuming and very resource-intensive.

Interestingly, New Zealand recently carried out a risk assessment of its use of rendered feedstuff for cattle. Its conclusion, supported by public consultation, was that since New Zealand had no cases of BSE among cattle and had very effective import controls, the use of a low-temperature rendering process for the production of cattle feed should continue. Public support for this approach demonstrates a very different response to that seen in the UK—though it should be borne in mind that a much greater proportion of New Zealand's population is involved in agriculture.

In Australia, the Commonwealth (i.e. the National government) is responsible for carrying out risk assessments but 'control and use' legislation is the responsibility of individual states. This means, of course, that the assessment of a risk is very effectively separated from the policy process associated with risk control. As a result, risk assessments in Australia are usually published at a national level without reference to ministers.

An important common authority is the Australian and New Zealand Food Agency (ANZFA). This operates on lines very similar to those proposed for the UK Food Standards Agency. It is managed by a Board and a Chief Executive Officer (CEO) and advises independently of ministers. The agency operates through a series of internal project teams, each working on a particular issue. A project team will include external members as well as those employed by the Agency. These external members may be scientific experts, or stakeholder, consumer, or lay representatives. For any issue likely to lead to new regulations or statutory change, there is a statutory requirement for two rounds of public consultation. There is consultation on other issues considered to have a significant public interest, e.g. development and use of genetically modified organisms. Because Australia does not have standing advisory committees, ANZFA may include individual experts as part of a project team or, for more complex issues, set up an *ad hoc* panel with relevant expertise.

Once an assessment has been published, it is up to the individual states to develop their own policy in relation to regulatory control and use. This model may give some indication of how risk assessment may become separated from policy development in the UK. Responsibility for assessment of risk is beginning to move from individual countries to a European forum, with member states then having to develop their own regulatory policy (although indications are that member states in the EU will have less freedom to develop their own policies than do individual states in Australia).

Experience in both Australia and New Zealand has shown that one consequence of carrying out a wide consultation on an important or sensitive issue is to make it very difficult for government to pursue a policy that is not supported by the consultation exercise.

For example, the Australian government wanted to set up a High Temperature Incinerator (HTI) for organic waste. A site was suggested, which led to a huge public outcry from those living in the area. As a result, an independent expert panel was set up which involved no government officials. This panel consulted widely and held public meetings across the country, including many rural areas. Its recommendation was that there was no support for HTIs. The wide consultation left the government little alternative but to accept the recommendation. The government then set up another consultation process amongst stakeholders, with Commonwealth and State officials acting as observers only. This time the remit was to come up with a solution for the disposal of the waste. The result was that stakeholders with very different interests began to work together to find an acceptable solution. With hindsight, the government recognizes this to be a much better solution for Australia than the original proposal for HTIs.

Though such success stories cannot be guaranteed, the case demonstrates that public participation can be extremely useful not only for gathering opinion but, if included in the decision-making process, for helping to achieve consensus and develop creative solutions. In general, the experience of countries which make considerable use of public participation in the risk analysis process is that it does offer some important advantages. These include the ability to achieve consensus and minimize adverse public and media reaction. People are reportedly much happier with the process, and the end result may be to find a better solution by taking account of a wider set of perspectives, including public perceptions. Where people are involved in the decision-making process, they are also more inclined to take responsibility for the outcome. These benefits translate into greater public trust of government and risk regulators.

Nevertheless, some disadvantages need to be carefully considered. Not only is the process very resource-intensive (with consequent financial implications) but it is also extremely slow and cumbersome. It should also be remembered that a wide consultation does effectively bind government to the recommendations of the exercise. This may be of particular concern if the recommendation is for a particularly expensive option.

## Summary

As the British advisory system on risk issues moves towards greater transparency and opens the development of risk management options to wider input, it is important to learn from the experience of others who have already moved some way down this road. Clearly there are difficulties to be overcome, not least the need for a significant 'cultural shift' on the part of regulators, politicians, the media, and the public if change is to lead to not only a more open process but also to better and more effective risk regulation and control. It is apparent from the variety of remits of the different expert advisory committees that what may be appropriate for one committee may not be so for another. This highlights the need for the role of each committee to be clearly defined, so that appropriate ways of making their work more transparent and open to public scrutiny can be followed. Careful thought is already being given to establishing more effective and open methodologies for assessing risks and developing the right policies to deal with them. While increased public participation will certainly have a greater role to play, the time and resources potentially involved make it important to try to identify the most appropriate models for dealing with particular types of risk issues. There are many different models, including focus groups, public hearings, consensus conferences, citizen advisory committees, citizens' juries, negotiated rule making, public opinion surveys, and even referenda (plus may other customized models), some described in the previous chapter. So far, however, particular approaches appear to have been adopted on an *ad hoc*, almost random basis. There is little or no evidence in the literature of systematic evaluation of the relative effectiveness of particular models for different situations (Rowe and Frewer 1998). Most reports of public participation also relate to a single, location-specific issue: such situations may have a very different dynamic to issues relating to broader government regulatory policy.

## REFERENCES

Office of Science and Technology (1997). *The use of scientific advice in policy making.* Office of Science and Technology, London, UK.

Interdepartmental Liaison Group on Risk Assessment (1998). *Risk communication: a guide to regulatory practice.* Interdepartmental Liaison Group on Risk Assessment, London, UK.

Smith, W. (1997). *Review of expert panels for provision of scientific and technical advice for development of public policy.* Ministry of Research Science and Technology (MORST), Auckland, New Zealand.

Rowe, G. and Frewer, L. J. (1998). *Public participation methods: a framework for evaluation.* Institute for Food Research, Reading, UK.

# PART 4

## Pulling the threads together

### Preface to Part 4

The aim of this final part of the book is to pull together some common themes and explore their practical implications. Given the range of contributors so far, one might expect this to be a tall order. Certainly there are areas of disagreement, and we ourselves would offer different interpretations of some of the specific events discussed. That is only to be expected. More importantly, there do seem to be some significant 'islands of agreement'—if not on an ideal destination then at least on the required direction of travel. For example, there seems to be some consensus around three principles that have been stressed within the Department of Health of late:

- while public reactions to risk can seem surprising, they are not totally unpredictable;
- effective risk communication is necessarily a two-way process;
- good risk communication requires a coherent strategy, rather than just *ad hoc* reaction to events.

These are offered only as a starting point. They may not be sufficient conditions for progress, but they do at least seem necessary. The following chapters explore the implications of these and other principles for the practice of risk communication. They are addressed particularly to those within organizations having to communicate about risks, whose reaction may otherwise be: 'yes, but what can we actually *do*?' It should also be clear that responsibility for 'doing something' runs much wider than those formally charged with a communication function. Indeed, some earlier contributors question whether 'communication' is a helpful term: for some, it still suggests a one-way process of information release. We disagree, but acknowledge the significance of the perception. Our own view reflects that now being propounded by the FAO and World Health Organization as a basic 'Principle of Risk Management':

'Ongoing reciprocal communication among all interested parties is an integral part of the risk management process. Risk communication is more than the dissemination of information, and a major function is the process by which information and opinion essential to effective risk management is incorporated into the decision'.

Report of the FAO/WHO Consultation on Risk Management 1997.

Taken seriously, this has profound implications. In particular, it means that everyone involved in risk assessment and management needs to attend to the issues raised by communication, both inward and outward. It also means that those with responsibility for organizational design, or with influence on the structure of institutions, need to take note. Even more widely, if trust 'when the crunch comes' depends on what impression people have of how the organization as a whole behaves, on how responsive it seems, and on the impression people have gained of it in dealing with otherwise quite unrelated matters—in short, on the elusive quality of reputation— these issues are indeed everyone's business.

# 16 Risk communication as a decision process

Peter Bennett, David Coles, and Anne McDonald
*Department of Health*

## Introduction

As can be seen from other chapters, it is all too easy to track the consequences of failure in risk communication: warnings that fail to warn (or cause unforeseen panic), reassurances that fail to reassure, and a general lack of trust all round. Nevertheless, it seems clear that some episodes are managed more effectively than others, and that this can have a cumulative impact. There is no justification for presuming that messages will always be misunderstood or disbelieved, *and that nothing can be done to mitigate this.* This chapter starts the process of pulling together the themes explored throughout the book in a form that can be used to guide good organizational practice. The aim is to provide a self-contained overview, while noting several issues explored in more depth in the remaining chapters below.

A key message of this volume as a whole is that risk communication is about much more than choice of words and numbers. Of course these are still vitally important—and the source of much angst, confusion, and recrimination. So formulating the message and presenting it effectively remains essential, but only as part of the overall effort. Risk management that overlooks stakeholders' basic concerns cannot usually be saved by good communication techniques late in the day—though much effort can still be brought low by a 'killer headline'.

Good practice therefore demands attention to two interlinked processes:

(1) the internal process of identifying issues, planning how to deal with them, taking action, and monitoring results;

(2) that of managing external relations—setting up consultation, engaging with other interested parties, etc.

This chapter offers some commentary on these processes before making some points about words, numbers, and their delivery. Finally, we consider some ways of embedding attention to these issues into organizational practice. The stress is on seeing all these as areas for decision-making. Whether in deciding what priority to give an issue, who to consult, or what words to use, choices made by default—'the way we always do it'—are still choices. They will be appropriate only by good fortune. However, we cannot offer a *recipe* for good practice. There is no one 'correct' way of managing a typical risk communication episode: the need is rather to be aware of the (broadly defined) risks and opportunities of different ways forward and to strike an informed balance.

At a higher level again, considering risk communication takes us into the realms of organizational (and institutional) design. This much is clear from the contributions to Part 3 above. This chapter is aimed primarily at establishing pointers to good practice within a given institutional structure. But if structures inhibit good practice, continued failures in risk communication may be one price paid for not considering the wider issues.

# Toward better processes

## Scanning, prioritizing, and preparation

Crisis conditions—combining time pressure, unexpectedness, and high levels of threat—almost always militate against effective decision-making. One defence is to ensure that effective procedures are in place in advance—the art of crisis planning. A simple example is to have a prepared list of the key actors liable to be involved in a specific type of risk issue, and actions needed to engage with them. Another defence against crisis is to spot possible difficulties in advance. The aim should therefore be to scan ahead, identifying possible risk issues and the communication challenges they may pose. In some cases the timing may be reasonably certain (for example, a report on a particular issue may be due to appear two months hence), in others much less so. Nevertheless, effective scanning requires attention to communication issues early on. This is one of several reasons (others are discussed below and in Chapter 9) to avoid treating communication as an 'add-on' to risk assessment, to be considered only once the other decisions have been made.

At minimum, scanning ahead should provide greater opportunity for *internal* consultation as to how emergent issues can be managed, between actors who may include policy leads, managers, administrators, technical experts, medical staff, communications professionals, and others. The 'cast list' will vary between organizations and across cases, but it can be guaranteed that everyone will have their own perspective. Differences in viewpoint can be used constructively to foster a broader view of the issues. Mismanaged, they provide sources both of internal resentment (on the part of those who feel unjustifiably ignored), and of confusing and contradictory public messages. The damage caused to external credibility by poor internal coordination is difficult to overstate.

Effective scanning will usually identify many potential issues, not all of which can (or should) be given equal attention. The findings outlined in Part 1 can be used to set risk communication priorities, alongside scientific assessment of the risks themselves. The 'fright factors' and 'media triggers' introduced in Chapter 1 can be used in simple checklists (see for example that reproduced in Fig. 16.1), or ideas taken from some of the more sophisticated approaches discussed in other chapters—e.g. on different dimensions of trust. The balance between different concerns will vary from organization to organization, depending on its role regarding the risks in question. No scanning approach can hope to spot all the relevant issues in advance: there will always be a need to firefight. In that context too, however, it should be possible to provide a rough-but-rapid diagnosis of *which* events carry the greatest danger of spiralling out of control. Even if precise predictions are not possible, there is no need to be routinely surprised by responses to messages about risks.

## What are the aims and who are the stakeholders?

Treating communication as a series of decisions *should* immediately trigger one key question in any specific case: *what are we trying to achieve?* As French and Maule point out in Chapter 19, this question is frequently *not* asked explicitly, and decision-making is consequently the poorer. Formulating specific objectives in turn requires a clear view of who the relevant *stakeholders* are—in the sense of those who are both affected by the issue and whose actions will have some effect on what happens. Who exactly is it hoped to influence and in what ways? Further thought may suggest that the intention may vary (for example, one may wish to warn some stakeholders and inform or reassure others). The very exercise of listing stakeholders and how they might or might not react can be highly informative in clarifying one's own aims: as noted later, it can also be expanded into more or less elaborate scenario-building exercises. The basic point is that one way or another, communication should relate to choices. Whether the aim is to explain one's own decisions, influence other actors or both, the connection needs to be clear. Otherwise a quite justifiable response to information about a risk is 'so what?'—what are you doing about it, and what am I supposed to do?

# COMMUNICATING ABOUT RISKS TO PUBLIC HEALTH: CHECKLIST OF KEY POINTS

1. This list can be used:
   - for **scanning** to help identify difficult cases
   - to guide reaction to **unforeseen incidents.**

## Anticipating public impact

2. **Responses are influenced by fright factors** and **media triggers** (see boxes). A high score on either list indicates a need for particular care. A high score on *both* should alert you to a possible high-profile scare. Conversely, it will be difficult to direct attention to low-scoring risks.

3. **'Indirect' effects** are commonly caused by people's responses to the original risk. Have possible economic, social, and political consequences been considered?

## Planning a communication strategy

4. Are the **aims** of communicating clear? Note that objectives should be:
   - agreed internally between relevant staff with different responsibilities (e.g. policy leads, technical advisors, press staff)
   - reviewed as the situation develops

5. Who are the **key stakeholders**? These will usually include both *intended* audiences and others who may react. What *other issues* may affect their actions?

6. What is known about **how different stakeholders perceive the issue**? What are the likely levels of **trust**, and what can be done to influence trust?

7. Can the proposed message be seen as **inconsistent with previous messages** or with other policies? How can this be avoided or, failing that, explained?

8. Are mechanisms in place for keeping all the above **under review?**

## The process of communication

9. Is there a checklist of **who to involve** at each stage of information release?

10. In deciding how and when to involve external stakeholders:
    - are decisions being considered as early as possible, and taken on a consistent and defensible basis?
    - are any **decisions against openness** both necessary and clearly explained?
    - have mechanisms for involvement been **made clear to others**?

11. **What other actions are being taken** to deal with the risk? Do these support or undermine the intended communication? What overall impression is being conveyed?

## Content of communication

12. Do statements attend to likely **values of the audiences** (e.g. perceived fairness or need to vent anger), as well as providing factual information? Is the emotional tone appropriate to this?

13. Have **uncertainties** in scientific assessments been acknowledged?

14. In any statements about **probabilities**:
    - if **relative risks** are given, is the 'baseline' risk clear?
    - do any **risk comparisons** serve to illuminate alternative options? Could any comparisons appear unfair or flippant?

15. Have **framing effects** of wording (e.g. 'lives lost' versus 'lives saved') been considered?

## Monitoring of decisions and outcomes

16. Are procedures in place to **monitor** actions and results?

17. Are there mechanisms for **reviewing** strategy and outcomes, and **disseminating** lessons for future practice?

## Further analysis

18. Might **further analysis** be appropriate? If so, has assistance been sought?

## Fright Factors

The following *perceptions* will make a risk seem less acceptable/more worrying

– risk is **involuntary**

– risk seen as **inequitable**

– risk seen as **inescapable**

– source of risk **unfamiliar or novel**

– risk **man-made** rather than natural

– **hidden and irreversible damage**

– danger to **small children** or **future generations**

– form of harm arouses **much dread**

– victims **identifiable**, not anonymous

– risk appears **poorly understood** by science

– **contradictory statements** from responsible sources

## Media Triggers

A story will be more newsworthy the more the following can be made to feature:

– Questions of **blame**

– Alleged **secrets and cover-ups**

– **Human interest**

– Links with existing **high-profile issues (or personalities)**

– **Conflict**

– **Signal value** (*"What next ?"*)

– **Many people at risk**, even if at low levels (*"It could be you !"*)

– **Visual impact**

– Story links to **sex** and/or **crime**

– **Snowballing** of reportage (*"A story because it's a story"*)

**Fig. 16.1** Risk communication checklist, Department of Health.

The term 'stakeholder' is used to direct attention more widely than just the *audience* for communication. Though knowing the intended audience(s) is important, the effects of communication can impact more widely— potentially on all those having to deal either with the risk itself or with the consequences of other people's responses. This is the territory of 'indirect effects' and social amplification of risks mapped out in Chapter 5. Politicians and the media are inevitably stakeholders in any major public health issue. So too are the public—seldom as a homogeneous mass, but differentiated according to who is more or less *at risk* and who is more or less exercised by an (established or alleged) hazard. But the list is usually much longer: relevant stakeholders in a national public health issue might include general practitioners, pharmacists, clinical specialists, charities, and campaigning groups—e.g. representing consumers, environmental lobbies, or those suffering particular forms of illness—various government departments and agencies, businesses, particular groups of scientists, the British Medical Association, local authorities, and so on. Many issues also have strong international or European dimensions—as seen earlier in several of the case-study chapters. It is therefore essential to consider, as early as possible, what responses from such actors would be welcome or harmful. This is so whether or not particular stakeholders are to be brought into the policy process through consultation or negotiation. If not, considering their possible responses can still help avoid pitfalls, e.g. the announcement held up due to last-minute legal objections. More importantly, a decision in favour of wider participation will not make it simply happen. Involving other stakeholders needs more forward thinking than is often recognized.

## Consultation and constructive engagement

Seriously attempting to communicate 'with' rather than 'at' people offers two distinct benefits. The first is in helping to establish trust—a point already emphasized consistently enough to need no repetition here. In this context, openness most obviously implies a presumption in favour of disclosing information (otherwise, reasons need to be given clearly and early). But more is usually needed than one-way information release. Stakeholders need to have as much opportunity as possible to *contribute*: those perceiving themselves to have been ignored or belittled will respond with antagonism even to 'full disclosure'. (Genuine reasons for lack of consultation—e.g. in responding rapidly to an emergency—are more likely to be respected if there is a track record of consulting when it *is* feasible.) In short, trust requires mechanisms to be in place for *listening to* potential audiences.

This brings us to the second potential benefit. Listening may be 'nice',[1] but there is also the chance of actually hearing something worthwhile! As a minimum, one may find out more as to why people out there are concerned (or not) about particular risks. But beyond that, they may have significant contributions to make toward dealing with the issue in hand, in particular in fostering a broader view.

## Contingency planning and 'assumption busting'

Research on public perceptions of risk is neatly complemented by studies of its organizational mismanagement. Large-scale failures have been studied in contexts as diverse as warfare, corporate policy, public-sector planning, international relations, and engineering. The psychological phenomenon of 'expert overconfidence' was noted in Chapter 1. The general point is that able decision-makers (and their advisers) can become fixed on a particular set of assumptions. Uncertainties are assumed away and alternative views ignored despite evidence that should have given pause for thought (Turner and Pidgeon 1997; Huxham and Dando 1981). These effects can be amplified when work is carried out in highly cohesive groups (Janis 1972). When trouble finally strikes no alternative plans are in place: commitments already made may be costly or impossible to undo and crisis ensues.

It is therefore essential to have ways of uncovering uncertainties and considering alternative scenarios so that responses can be considered in outline. For example, the scientific evidence on risks may itself be subject to significant uncertainties—as many other contributors have stressed. But acknowledging this often flies in the face of demands for certainty from public and policy-makers alike. Policy-makers may be tempted to use science as a totem with which to ward off criticism. For the public, failure to deliver certainty can fuel the cynical belief that anything can be 'proven'. There is thus massive pressure for premature closure of debate.

While acknowledging uncertainty is never easy, greater damage can be caused both by premature dogmatism and by failure to consider different scenarios—even if only in private. If an initial public position has to be modified, preparedness will limit the damage by allowing change to be both prompt and convincingly explained. The key to preparedness is determined 'assumption-busting' early on, so as to identify the most critical suppositions. One form of contingency planning is to ask '*what if* the key scientific evidence were thrown into doubt?'. Clues as to which assumptions to vary can be found by looking critically at the 'pedigree' of key evidence—how it

---

1. c.f. 'All we need to do is to be nice to them'—a stage about halfway up (or down) Fischhoff's (1995) ladder of developmental stages in risk communication.

was generated and by whom (Funtowicz and Ravetz, 1990). But sometimes even the highest pedigree assumptions turn out to be mistaken. As Maxwell (Chapter 7) argues in the context of the BSE crisis, there is a need to look at non-orthodox views. The point is *not* that all views should somehow be accorded equal weight. Despite the attractions of a romantic, 'they said Copernicus was mad' view of science, most dissident views remain just that. But that should not stop one asking the questions: '*what if* the accepted view is mistaken?'. What would be the consequences for what we are saying now? Can we still give a clear message while not giving too many hostages to fortune?

While it is possible (and desirable) to carry out assumption-busting in private, an open process should help. Those coming to the situation with a different perspective can prevent a too-easy consensus and may raise the 'obvious question' that turns out not to be so obvious.

Another area for contingency planning is to consider different ways in which an issue could be framed by the media, while satisfying the need for a good story. This can help clarify possible responses and suggest what might influence choices of storyline. The key question might be something as simple as 'are we to be seen as part of the problem or part of the solution?'.

## Monitoring and review

Finally, each communication episode—successful or otherwise—represents an opportunity for organizational learning. This will only occur if there are mechanisms to ensure that the reasons for decisions are logged and outcomes noted. Given pressures on time, procedures need to work with as little additional effort as possible—data recorded *at the time* being of particular value. Review should then be undertaken as a matter of course— rather than *post mortems* being triggered only by perceived failures. The main aim should be to identify learning points of possible future relevance, and these need to be shared with staff in other relevant policy areas. The results should then feed into routine analysis of new issues. In this way, collective experience may be put to best use (Chapters 19 and 20).

# Words, numbers and delivery

## Background

Treating risk communication as a two-way process in no way makes more traditional communication skills redundant. Choice of words and numbers for particular audiences, clarity and style of delivery, and attention to the 'mechanics' of public announcements all remain essential. Much has been written on communication in general (Thomas and Lilford 1995), and we take the fundamentals as read. There are, however, some additional factors involved in communicating about risks to public health. Some basic points about risk perceptions should be part of the 'mental furniture' of anyone involved in risk communication—and in risk analysis more generally. The following summarize points noted in Chapter 1 and illustrated in several different contexts in the intervening chapters.

1. People usually judge messages first according to the trustworthiness of the source, and only second according to content.

2. Perceived risk has many dimensions which cannot be expressed on a single scale such as probable number of fatalities: hence the importance of 'fright factors', etc.

3. There may well be a general tendency to overstate the occurrence of rare events.

4. Disagreements are typically about both facts and values, and perceptions of specific risks linked to wider beliefs. 'Facts' about one risk in isolation may therefore have little impact.

5. Messages about risk will be picked up and interpreted by many audiences, not just those intended.

6. The behaviour of those influenced by the message will impact on other people and modify their behaviour in turn ('indirect effects', 'social amplification').

7. There are identifiable factors which will tend to make a risk issue into a good story.

On the last topic, a more extended account of the relationships between the political system, the media, and public beliefs is provided in Chapter 18.

## The key message

Looking now at the specifics of outward communication, the first point is to refer back to objectives. In particular, there needs to be a decision as to the *main* intended message, stated in simple terms. Some practitioners refer to this as a SOCHO—Single, Over-riding Communication Health Objective (c.f. Murphy 1997). There can also be a few subsidiary messages, and fuller versions of arguments and evidence should be available—with uncertainties duly acknowledged—for those who wish to pursue them. But the priority must be clear. Where there is some complex science to convey, formulating a SOCHO without doing violence to it—and without giving a false impression of certainty—is difficult. (It may be helpful to consider possible headlines about actions rather than about the magnitude of a risk *per se*). The alternative, however, is much worse. If it is difficult to simplify the message, the answer cannot be to leave others to make of it what they will.

As noted in Chapter 1, there are always alternative ways of framing an issue—of arranging the elements into some coherent picture. Of course, framing is often contested: other actors will want to promote their own interpretation of events, and they may succeed. This is a legitimate part of debate. Nevertheless, deciding on the key *intended* message is a start. It will also be helpful to have some idea of audiences' existing framing of the issue in question—e.g. from survey results. Would the intended message reinforce this (providing new information that would easily 'fit in') or challenge it? If the latter, what can be said or done to help trigger a change in view? To ask such questions is not to reduce communication to mere spin-doctoring. In the present context, manipulation of framing is arguably unethical and probably impractical. The main need is rather to avoid accidental mismatches in framing, either because the possibility has not been considered or because too little is known about public perceptions. Consultation will again generally help in this respect, as may small-scale piloting of messages (perhaps as an internal exercise) or brainstorming workshops.[2]

Finally, formulating the key message should also prompt a check on whether the organization's overall behaviour is actually compatible with it. If not, at least one needs to change! For example, if the intended message is of 'urgent investigation', is this demonstrably happening? Alternatively, is the message 'don't panic' being delivered by an organization taking what look like desperate measures?

## Language and science

Aside from the general requirements of clarity of expression, etc., there are three specific challenges in translating scientific results into messages for public consumption. The first two have to do with conceptions of cause-and-effect.

1. Many scientific results will be couched in terms of aggregate populations. The public will primarily be concerned with risks to individuals.

---

2. A further possibility (not so far tried, to our knowledge) would be to use the typology of cultural theory to help generate alternative ways of framing issues. In other words, one could ask 'what would be an extreme individualist's response to this? A pure egalitarian's? . . .' and so on. This in turn could suggest forms of argument to support the intended message more effectively for each type.

2.  Scientists will tend to reject a suggested causal link for which there is no positive evidence (c.f. Chapter 3). The public will require strong proof *against* a link that looks intuitively plausible.

These differences cannot be resolved simply by insisting that the scientific viewpoint is the correct one. The second, in particular, has led to widespread dissatisfaction with the formula of 'there is no evidence that ...' X causes a risk of Y. (There is a case for avoiding the phrase 'there is no evidence that ...' altogether, unless prefaced by the word 'although'.)

A more constructive approach would be (a) to acknowledge the face-value plausibility of a link, (b) to point out the evidence one would expect to find if the link existed, and (c) to show how serious investigation has not found such evidence. If (b) or (c) cannot be provided, then 'no evidence' is anyway a dubious reassurance. Even if they can, persuasiveness is not guaranteed. A cup of plausibility can be worth a bucket of statistics—sometimes, it should be noted, for scientists too.

The third point has to do with emotional tone.

3.  Scientific results are generally and quite properly couched in dry, unemotional language. This alienates an audience that is frightened, outraged, or both.

As Taig argues in Chapter 17, bridging this gap may be particularly difficult for government and the public sector. The need to show empathy with emotion applies not only to language but to style of delivery: a cool, detached demeanour may *feel* 'professional' but is all too easily *perceived* as uncaring or arrogant. If emotions are running high, effective communication will mean addressing these *first*.

## Probabilities as numbers

We offer two specific points about the use of numbers in risk communication; as with the use of words these are in addition to more universal points, e.g. those in Huff's (1954) classic *How to lie with statistics*.

1.  Numerical comparisons between different risks should be used only with extreme caution.

The pitfalls in this area to be so severe that one leading source carries a repeated 'health warning': USE OF THESE COMPARISONS CAN SERIOUSLY DAMAGE YOUR CREDIBILITY (Covello *et al.* 1988). As noted in Chapter 1, it is helpful to compare like with like (e.g. voluntary risk with voluntary), and any use of comparisons to imply *acceptability* should be avoided. If the aim is to aid understanding of rough orders of magnitude, familiar comparators such as 'about one person in a small town' for '1 in 10 000' (Calman and Royston 1997) may be more helpful than comparing different risks directly. Comparisons with irrelevant risks—particularly if trust is already lacking—may be seen as sophistry or special pleading. Above all, flippant comparisons—which seem both to trivialize the risk and patronize the audience—are to be avoided.

The second point has to do with statements about relative risks—changes over time or differences between groups:

2.  In any statement about relative risks, the baseline risk must be made clear and its significance explained.

Because relative risks make attractive media copy, it will also be helpful to anticipate *other people's* use of such statistics, and to have ready ways of putting them in perspective. Taken out of context, relative risks can seriously mislead, directing attention toward smaller absolute risks at the expense of greater ones.

## Embedding better practice

If the points set out so far are accepted—at least in broad outline—what can organizations actually *do* to improve risk communication at a 'systemic' level? The answers are many and various—not least because organizations themselves differ in structure and culture, have different responsibilities, and start with different problems. However, it seems appropriate to conclude this chapter by outlining a programme of work within the Department of Health, in progress since the summer of 1996. This may be of interest both because of the Department's inevitable position as a major player in debates about risks to public health, and because it illustrates some types of activity that can be undertaken in many settings. Note the reference to *a* programme of work, not *the* programme. Much else of relevance is happening within the Department and among the expert committees that advise government (see Chapters 11, 15). Within the National Health Service much is also being done at regional level and by individual Health Authorities and Trusts. Indeed, it is encouraging to find broadly similar conclusions coming from that direction (Zimmern 1997; Chapter 8), and similarly from the inter-departmental studies, e.g. that already outlined in Chapter 9 (see also ILGRA 1998).

There are two generic ways of assisting with decisions:

•  bringing to bear substantive knowledge
•  assisting with the decision process.

On the first, there is clearly no shortage of literature on risk perception and communication—as evidenced by Part 1 of this volume. The challenge is to summarize relevant findings without doing too much violence to the underlying research or implying that the results are more clear-cut than they really are. On the second, disciplines such as operational research (management science) offer various problem-structuring methods—for example, scenario-building, stakeholder analysis, classification of uncertainties—that can be used to guide discussion of specific cases. These can be used in a fairly simple way to promote 'structured brainstorming', or developed into more elaborate analysis. Setting up facilitated workshops involving staff with responsibilities for different aspects of the case can help bring different perspectives to bear and improve coordination.

With this in mind—and acknowledging that there is unlikely to be one single key to success—the programme within the Department has had four linked elements:

1.  *General guidance* on risk communication has been provided through a booklet summarizing relevant research and offering suggestions on the communication process. The topics covered loosely match Chapter 1 of this volume and the earlier sections of this chapter. Its content evolved in response to comment from both inside and outside the Department, a process itself probably helping to focus interest and awareness. The result was circulated in late 1997 as a Departmental booklet (Department of Health 1997) and reprinted in early 1998. An even more condensed aid has been the checklist of key points shown previously in Fig. 16.1. This is incorporated into the booklet and also used as a free-standing item. Serving as a common point of reference for all the other elements in the programme, the checklist has been successively refined through use in developmental workshops, case studies, and decision-support exercises outlined below.

2.  *Developmental workshops* are described more fully by French and Maule in Chapter 19. These events are designed to develop participants' ability to identify and manage risk communication issues. Guided by facilitators, staff work on fictional but realistic cases, structured so as to bring out points of particular interest. The aim is both to promote personal learning and to indicate possible improvements to Departmental practice.

3.  *Case-study seminars* are based on discussions of past cases, involving members of staff with significant responsibility for managing them. At each event the handling of the case in question and the current guidance are evaluated against each other (using a version of the checklist reworded to form a 'protocol' for enquiring about past episodes). Lessons have been drawn from each case and the guidelines themselves progressively refined. The typical format is of individual interviews with case-providers,

circulation of a background paper based on these, an informal seminar, and then a final report. The case studies complement other efforts, both internal (e.g. reviews of food hazard incidents) and cross-governmental.

4. *Decision Support* has been undertaken to underpin handling of various live issues, e.g. through decision-support workshops. As a minimum all interventions have made use of the checklist to structure discussion. Some have also employed specific idea-management methods, e.g. using post-its and flipcharts to generate and structure key uncertainties, or brainstorming different scenarios. In each case the aim has been to clarify the objectives and possible handling options, set out key stakeholders, how they may respond and how one might engage with them, and to form contingency plans to cope with the most important uncertainties. This helps the group gauge the advantages and disadvantages of different communication approaches. Opportunities can also be set up for later review of the case to help establish learning points.

# Final comments

The programme just outlined has been intended to raise awareness of relevant research and to promote earlier and more systematic attention to risk communication research. At the same time, we have tried to avoid any impression of peddling easy answers. We have been able to facilitate joint working on various risk issues, and a portfolio of real cases analysed in real time is gradually accumulating, raising the possibilities for cumulative organizational learning. In some cases where the programme has not had direct input, the underlying ideas are reported to have had some influence. We could not expect these relatively small-scale efforts to have a revolutionary effect, but they may be contributing to an overall change in climate.

## REFERENCES

Calman, K. C. and Royston, G. (1997). Risk language and dialects. *British Medical Journal*, **313**, 799–802.

Covello, V. T., Sandman, P. M. and Slovic, P. (1988). *Risk communication, risk statistics and risk comparisons: a manual for plant managers*. Chemical Manufacturers' Association, Washington DC.

Department of Health (1997). *Communicating about risks to public health: pointers to good practice*. Department of Health, London.

Fischhoff, B. (1995). Risk perception and communication unplugged: twenty years of process. *Risk Analysis*, **15**, 137–45.

Funtowicz, S. O. and Ravetz, J. R. (1990). *Uncertainty and quality in science for policy*. Kluwer, Dordrecht.

Huff, D. (1954). *How to lie with statistics*. Gollancz. Reprinted in 1973 by Penguin.

Huxham, C. S. and Dando, M. R. (1981). Is bounded-vision an adequate explanation of decision-making failures? *Omega*, **9**, 371–9.

ILGRA (1998). *Risk communication: a guide to regulatory practice*. Inter-departmental Liaison Group on Risk Assessment, Health and Safety Executive, London.

Janis, I. L. (1972). *Victims of groupthink*. Houghton-Mifflin, Boston.

Murphy, C. (1997). Talking to the media. *Public Health Laboratory Service Microbiology Digest*, **14**, 209–13.

Thomas, H. and Lilley, R. (1995). *If they haven't heard it, you haven't said it! A guide to better communication*. LGC Communications, London.

Turner, B. A. and Pidgeon, N. F. (1997). *Man-made disasters* (2nd edn) Butterworth-Heinemann, Oxford.

Zimmern, R. (1997). *Chance and choice: annual report of the Director of Public Health*. Cambridge and Huntingdon Health Authority, Cambridge.

# 17 Risk communication in government and the private sector: wider observations

Tony Taig
*Risk Solutions, AEA Technology*

## Introduction

This chapter offers some observations and conclusions on risk communication and public health based on two sources. The first is a recent substantial project on risk communication carried out on behalf of the Health and Safety Executive and a number of other UK government departments (Chapter 9). The second source is the author's wider experience in consulting in the public and private sectors on risk management and communication, largely outside the sphere of public health.

The observations relate to risk communication on public health in comparison with other public and private sector situations, and are grouped under four headings:

- common problems
- real advances
- science versus emotion
- scope and purpose of risk communication.

The observations are followed by some conclusions as to the similarities and differences of approach in the public and private sectors, and the challenges ahead for each.

## Common problems

In the course of a career largely spent applying concepts of risk in new areas, it has never been long before, in a new client organization, somebody has taken the author aside to let him know that 'you really must appreciate the absolutely *unique* difficulty in public communication associated with (the nuclear industry, electromagnetic fields, rail or aviation safety, food, health, water ...)'.

In fact the problems are usually very similar, and are founded in a lack of trust and confidence in risk information provided by 'experts', and in the processes by which decisions are made. It is very seldom that public concerns are based on an objective evaluation that risk is too high, or on suggestions that there are alternative risk control strategies available of demonstrably superior effectiveness. Instead, typical manifestations of the underlying problem of trust include:

(1) over-reaction or even panic when new information about risks is made public;

(2) difficulty in rejecting ineffective and expensive solutions to risk problems that have captured the public imagination;

(3) debate characterized by discussion of features of risk control measures, with little focus on their effectiveness in actually reducing or controlling risk itself;

(4) difficulty in advocating significant change in the 'recipe' for controlling risk, no matter how beneficial.

On the first of these, there has actually been very considerable progress in recent years. But the others remain really tough issues in both the public and the private sector. The third point is perhaps the most fundamental: 'risk reduction' is a very intangible benefit, which people are often asked to take on trust, whereas *the activities and things which control risk* tend to be much more tangible—airbags, fire extinguishers, lifebelts, hospitals, radar systems for air traffic control, a car to drive children to school instead of walking, etc. Trying to argue against an established preference for one risk control recipe over another thus requires a very fundamental shift of debate from a 'tangible features' to an 'intangible benefits' plane. Real trust between the parties is an absolute prerequisite for any such debate.

## Real advances

While the commonality of problems may be cause for gloom, there are also some favourable indications that the opportunity for real debate about risk —to find solutions to problems which will help raise quality of life while making that higher quality more accessible and affordable for the many, not just for the few—is increasing steadily. Four examples are considered here.

First, there is massive growth of *interest in and awareness of* risk as an important topic. This can be seen not only in the attention paid to unpleasant risk issues in the media, but also in an increasing tendency for the private sector and the marketplace to use risk as a key factor to differentiate themselves from others—whether in cars, investment plans, or in provision of different levels of service (with different prices) for different buyers.

Second, communication has been the subject of massive *research and practical development* over the past several decades. Areas such as crisis communications are no longer 'black arts' understood only by an elite few, but have become the theme for a large and successful subset of the PR and communications consulting 'industry'. Incidents such as the Perrier contamination and the Kegworth air crash have shown how the private sector has developed the means not only to address public concerns linked to a crisis, but also to demonstrate commitment to addressing those concerns. There is clear proof that trust and confidence can be built out of potentially crippling situations.

Third, there has been an explosion of *communications technology*, and with it the potential for massive social amplification of messages about risk —either negative or positive.

Fourth and finally, following the spate of major disasters in the mid-late 1980s, there have been some well-publicized 'test cases' that have *stimulated genuine public questioning* (albeit among a limited audience at present) of knee-jerk initiatives to do something large and visible about risks, only for it to be found later to be of very limited effectiveness. The major programme of removing wooden escalators from the London Underground following the King's Cross fire is a good example. There is a much more favourable climate for discussing the *effectiveness* of risk control measures today than at any time hitherto.

## Science versus emotion

One of the areas where government has differed most widely from the private sector has been in its relative lack of immediacy of interest in people's perceptions and attitudes, as opposed to 'scientific' hard facts. In the private sector it is axiomatic that perception is everything, and that perceptions can be changed either by changing the underlying product or service, or by managing perception while the goods remain unaltered. As a broad generalization, government seems very uneasy with this approach and, in its concern not to be seen as 'manipulating' opinion, frequently adopts approaches and behaviours which destroy trust and confidence.

As a framework to illustrate this point, consider the following simple axioms taught to the author some years ago as a 'rule of thumb' for communicating about risk. The framework has four simple elements, which are highly interlinked:

## 1. Emotion (or empathy)

As scientists, public health practitioners and experts tend deliberately to avoid allowing any hint of emotion to creep into their work or their voices in their anxiety to preserve objectivity. But to most listeners, the contest between a dry and unemotive speaker and one who appeals to the emotions is a very unequal one. The natural tendency of government in most debates about risk is to respond to concerns by going into facts. Government actions on risk issues generally take the form of controls which experts consider will reduce the risk. Such actions may (and probably often do) fail utterly to address the root of public concerns, which often have much more to do with emotional responses to people than with an objective judgement that risks are too high.

## 2. Concern

Many government announcements about risk exemplify a phenomenon which has also bedevilled many in the private sector. In their anxiety not to cause alarm, any information about a risk is immediately qualified with ten good reasons not to worry too much about it. This can all too easily create the impression that the risk has been dismissed as being of little concern, and thus that there is no chance that people's real concerns will be taken seriously. Respect for people's concerns (however irrational they might appear) is well proven to be a necessary foundation for building trust and confidence.

## 3. Commitment

It is vital to be committed, and to be able to demonstrate commitment, to effective management of risk. The point above about the intangibility of risk but the tangibility of risk controls is very relevant here—if we want to convince people that what 'we' have to say about risk has validity, we need to be able to demonstrate that 'we' are committed and able to deliver against our promises. To paraphrase former US President Jimmy Carter: if it were a crime to reduce risks to the public, would there be enough evidence to convict you?

## 4. Benefit

This is another area where both government and many involved in risk communication in the private sector can learn much from the marketplace.

One of the worst mistakes that can be made in advertizing or marketing is for the seller of goods to 'push' features to which they (the seller) attach great significance, but which the target customers do not appreciate—or worse, regard as irrelevant or even positively disadvantageous. If we want to convince people of a course of action we want to take, or tougher still to persuade them to change their own behaviour, it is vital to articulate the benefit *in terms relevant to them*. There is no point telling people a new control regime is better because it will save money for industry or government. On the other hand, greater affordability and accessibility of goods and services, or less exclusion of people at the margins (which often amount to very much the same thing), can be powerful 'selling' messages.

## Scope and purpose of risk communication

The final, and in my view most important, observation relates to the breadth of scope and purpose which applies to risk management and communication in government and in the private sector. This is illustrated in Fig. 17.1. There is a wide spectrum of types of activity included within 'communication', and their relative importance is different in government and in the private sector.

Whereas the private organization's primary concern is to protect itself and its customers from risk, the primary concern of government, as a regulator, is typically to protect others from the unwanted side-effects of markets meeting customer needs. With reference to Fig. 17.1, much of the private sector's communication tends to focus towards the top right of the figure, on understanding customer needs and on influencing people to buy at the right price. On the other hand, government tends to focus much of its energies towards the bottom left. It provides information to help consumers make well-informed choices (protecting them from market manipulation). Through regulation and enforcement, it also tells people what to do in a much more

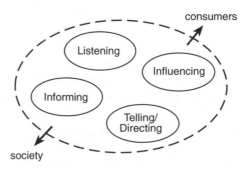

**Fig. 17.1**  Risk Communication: breadth of scope and purpose.

direct way than any private sector organization can. Given this difference, it is not surprising that government and the private sector have evolved different approaches to communication generally, and to risk communication in particular.

Nevertheless, just as the private sector is widening its focus to embrace a more holistic, 'stakeholder' approach to managing relationships with wider audiences, so government is increasingly recognizing the need for a wider approach to risk communication. Throughout the recent risk communication benchmarking project, people in government departments and agencies expressed massive interest in improving the effectiveness of risk communication in the 'listening', as well as the 'telling' mode, and in the importance of communication as a policy instrument in its own right to influence behaviour (where this is a valid policy objective). The overarching conclusion of the project was that communication is an integral part of risk management and policy. Whether identifying policy needs, developing policy objectives, planning how best to achieve them, implementing or evaluating policy initiatives, communication is instrumental at every stage, and a key determinant of effectiveness throughout. To regard risk communication as a 'bolt on' activity once everything has been resolved on the basis of 'science' is to lose a major opportunity.

Integration of risk communication and risk management must mean that *communication is able to influence and change the course of risk policy*. Those interested in and affected by risk policy have a very reasonable expectation that they should be involved in its determination. There are some excellent examples where this is the case, but many where it is not.

Experts are needed to assess risks, to assess the effectiveness of alternative approaches to risk control, and to predict the outcomes if we choose different ways forward. But the people affected have to be involved in making the value judgements about which of those outcomes are preferred.

The Chief Medical Officer is the right person to advise on the risks of eating beef on the bone, but has no competence to weigh people's rejection or acceptance of those risks against the value they attach to T-bone steak or their traditional roast rib. At the end of the day even the best communication from government to the public will fail unless it is matched by the means to enable public voices to be heard in, and to influence, public policy.

# Conclusions

To summarize, there are both some significant similarities and some important differences between the public and private sectors, and some common challenges faced by each.

There are similarities in that many of the important issues encountered in risk communication arise in both sectors, and there is a growing pool of expertise and experience that is available to, and used by, both. The contribution of government expertise and experience to that pool should not be underestimated.

There are significant differences in the degree to which what is already known is applied and implemented. Implementation of what is established is generally higher in the private sector (with some honourable exceptions in parts of government). Government sometimes seems to possess a remarkable capacity for research in this area but a very limited capacity to implement change using the results. There is an important cultural difference between public and private sectors in terms of their familiarity and comfort levels in dealing with issues of perception—critical in building trust and confidence. There is also the issue of scope and purpose of risk communication, where there are legitimate differences between public and private sectors, and there is significant interest within government in exploring the relevance of private sector techniques.

Finally, there are important challenges faced by both the public and the private sectors, which are extremely relevant to risk communication and public health. These are:

- to move from a 'bolt-on' to a more integrated approach to risk communication, and

- to progress towards real public involvement in determining public risk policy.

# 18 Risk communication: the relationships between the media, public beliefs, and policy-making

David Miller and Sally Macintyre
*Stirling Media Research Institute, Stirling University* and
*Director, MRC Medical Sociology Unit, Glasgow University*

## Introduction

Risk communication is a complex phenomenon which involves a large number of contending and cooperating institutions and corporations, media organizations, and a range of publics and policy, cultural and political outcomes. However, communicating risk is often examined from the vantage point of only one part of the 'circuit of communication' (Miller *et al.* 1998). Thus we find discussions of the mediation of specific risks (either in scientific/ bureaucratic fora or in the press and broadcast media), examinations of 'lay perspectives' or public opinion on risk, or attempts to evaluate risk communication to internal and external audiences of a particular organization. There are also discussions of risk communication in general. Some of the cruder arguments in either of these approaches tend to identify the 'problem' of risk communication as either poor communication skills on the part of experts, media sensationalism and irresponsibility, or public ignorance or hysteria. Such views do seem to have been somewhat discredited in recent years although they retain something of a foothold in academic, public, and policy debate (Miller 1995; Miller and Reilly 1995). Even more sophisticated arguments often tend to deal with differing parts of the circuit of communication in isolation or have unduly one-dimensional perspectives on particular moments in the circuit. We are thinking here of approaches which accept that the media cannot be wished away, but nevertheless tend to see the mass media in predominantly negative terms. Alternatively, some of the more sympathetic approaches to public or lay perceptions also suffer from an inability to understand the way in which information is assimilated by the public.

Our suggestion is that a wider view of the processes of risk communication is useful. We cannot understand the actual behaviour of experts, the media, or the public in isolation from each other. Instead these need to be examined in the context of their interactions. We suggest that we should look at the communication of public health risks in a more complex fashion, as the product of an interaction between four sets of actors:

1. Social and political institutions (including natural and social scientific research).
2. Media organizations.
3. The public.
4. Decision-makers.

The interaction between these actors constitutes what we call the circuit of communication. Our argument is firstly that each of the different elements of the circuit needs sustained analysis which is sensitive to variation as well as similarity (e.g. not an assumption that media coverage or public opinion is homogenous). There is a need to trace the differing pathways between different elements of the circuit. We need to ask not just what is said by risk communicators or the media or believed by the public, but why. In other words, there is a need to understand the dynamic relations between different elements of the circuit, as well as to study the content of the different moments of the circuit in order to build up a better picture.

If we see the relationship between these elements of the circuit as interactive and dynamic we can begin to understand the way in which issues rise and fall on the public agenda. Public issues emerge when there are political disputes about risk information, very often informed by disputes at the level of science (e.g. BSE, *Salmonella*, HIV/AIDS).

This way of examining risk communication also has a methodological implication, which is that the circuit of communication needs to be examined in a holistic way. Examining only part of the circuit directly runs the risk of over- or underplaying the importance of the area studied, or of other areas. Thus, to examine only public perceptions or the genesis of scientific advice, or the preparation of communication campaigns, misses the relations between the various moments of communication.

The size, scope, and length of issues on the public agenda do not mirror their objective severity measured in terms of human misery or death. But rather than bemoan this fact, it seems more productive to try and understand why this is the case.

# Social and political institutions

Without sources of information, there would be no news. Social and political institutions have a fundamental role in risk communication. This is true both in the sense that large bureaucracies produce significant amounts of information every day for use by a wide variety of audiences, (including the mass media), and in the sense that risk communication campaigns can involve direct communication with particular publics through the production of leaflets, posters, and advertizing materials. In both cases there are a number of factors that influence (a) the planning, and (b) the execution of risk communication strategies.

## Planning risk communication

There are a number of potential problems in putting together risk communication campaigns.

### Science

Getting to grips with the complexity of the science in relation to certain risks is always potentially tricky. Divisions between scientists can make unambiguous statements difficult. In practice there is a system of expert advisory committees but, as the case of BSE shows, the way in which scientific advice is extracted can be subject to claims and counter-claims about the massaging of science (Miller, 1999). It is also clear that the remit of scientific investigations and membership of committees can direct the kinds of answers that are reached (for example, an animal health versus a public health approach to BSE).

### Communicating science

Perhaps more importantly, the process of translating scientific advice into official reports, press releases, and health education campaigns is also potentially tricky since it brings all sorts of calculations about communication effectiveness into play. This can work in two ways. First, calculations about what the media or the public might make of particular statements are necessarily involved in risk communication, but this can be at the expense of accuracy, or of denying uncertainty, as in absolute statements between 1990 and 1995 about the lack of risk from BSE. Secondly, calculations about what is politically possible can also impinge on government attempts at risk communication. Perhaps the best known example here is the agonizing in the Department of Health (and wider in government) in 1985–7 about whether explicit AIDS information was politically, as well as medically, desirable (Miller *et al.* 1998).

Such problems are given greater complexity with the involvement of a wide range of different professionals in the production of risk information. This applies to media relations but can be even more crucial to health education material. For example, in the AIDS campaign a wide range of professional groupings were centrally involved (ministers, administrative civil servants, medical civil servants, information officers, market researchers, advertizers, health educators, expert advisors, etc.). Many of these groups had opposed conceptions of communication planning and effectiveness, as well as differing sensitivities as to what was politically possible. For example, some ministers were concerned about the explicitness of AIDS advertizing (as has been confirmed by the former Chief Medical Officer, Sir Donald Acheson (1992)). Furthermore, professional communicators who favoured fear-arousal campaigns and 'impact' in advertizing often clashed with health educators who favoured sensitivity and recommending positive alternatives to penetrative sex. Government officials and ministers tend to present risk communication as a technical process (Miller *et al*. 1998; Miller 1999). In practice it can involve a complex web of interlocking disputes and alliances, which sometimes results in the communication of messages that, as a result of compromises and political interventions, are contradictory, vague, or contain little useful information and with which none of those involved are satisfied (Miller *et al*. 1998). Similar professional conflicts have also been noted in the somewhat less politically sensitive area of communication on coronary heart disease (Farrant and Russell 1986).

## Executing risk communication strategies

Once the message is agreed, there are all sorts of further obstacles to surmount. These include competition with opposing interests in government, as well as with the wide range of other perspectives on offer in the media, and cooperation with other interests and the formation of alliances

### Competition within government

Risk communication strategies may be hampered by conflicting interests inside government, either within or between departments. This is especially the case if such interests 'go public' even in the minimal sense of 'off the record briefings'. We can point to the controversy over *Salmonella* enteritidis PT4 in 1988–1989 as such a case. This is not only important in that it indicates conflict in government, but because this in itself will become an added reason for media interest.

### Competition with other interests

The strategies formulated by social institutions for influencing the media and decision-making are forced to compete with those of other organizations (whether they be scientific establishments, government departments, business ventures, or pressure groups). This is important for two reasons. First, there can be a wide range of information available to the public with which risk communication activities have to compete. Health educators sometimes refer to this as 'background noise' to their own campaigns. But given the large amounts of money spent on commercial advertizing and the omnipresence of the news and entertainment media, the converse is more accurate. Furthermore, there is a variety of organizations engaged in risk communication, which may have diverging reasons for and interests in managing risk (e.g. to protect corporate reputation, increase sales, further campaigning demands, etc.). This is an inevitable part of our culture, and there is no intrinsic reason why information emanating from government should be believed above that provided by competing interests. One implication of this is that government is itself a player in competition for media space and public sympathy, rather than a neutral arbiter.

### Cooperation

Cooperation and the building of coalitions are also important in that a broad consensus in a particular policy arena makes risk communication much more likely to succeed. The coalition built around public health interests on AIDS in 1985–1989 is a key example of such effective cooperation (Miller *et al.* 1998).

The consequence of the discussion in this section is to suggest that many of the problems of risk communication are not simply attributable to the poor communicative skills of officials (although these exist), the reporting of the media, or public response. Instead, we would want to argue that sometimes these problems are attributable to government actions. However, it is in the context of the interaction of government with the other actors set out here that risk communication has its impact.

## Media organizations

Much discussion of risk communication tends to see the role of the media as a predominantly negative one. 'The media' are dismissed as an homogeneous bloc whose penchant for sensation and irresponsibility is an obstacle to rational risk communication. We would suggest that the media are neither uniform nor consistently negative. This latter point can be made in relation to both the particular interests of risk communicators in having their messages carried and in relation to the democratic role of the media.

Media institutions do pursue readers with a variety of crude and not so crude techniques. However, there are clear differences in the types of material that appear both within and between media. For example, specialist correspondents have a distinctive role on both broadsheet and mid-market tabloid papers. Medical and scientific reporters tend to be very knowledge-able about their areas of responsibility. This can mean both that they adopt an advocate role for key sources in the medical and scientific community and that they can spot news management activities by their sources more quickly than their non-specialist colleagues. Accordingly, their coverage will tend to differ from that of freelances or of political correspondents who are drafted in when the story becomes a bigger public issue. On occasions, specialists can be regarded as performing a positive role for the risk communicator. This role might also (coincidentally) be regarded as positive for the public interest. One key area in which the bulk of the broadcast media and many newspapers (especially their specialists in medicine, science, and health) operated in a positive way from the point of view of government risk communicators was AIDS. Here the official message on heterosexual trans-mission was overwhelmingly supported (notwithstanding an active cam-paign against this by some newspapers) by the bulk of the media (especially broadcasting) and was very effective in convincing the public (Miller *et al.* 1998).

However, the public interest and the interest of the risk communicator are not always the same thing and there may be occasions where specialist reporters are perceived as promoting the sectional interests of their sources. Mediating such issues is the editorial hierarchy, which can on occasion result in conflict between the editorial priorities of the paper and those of the specialist.

Science tends to make front-page news when scientific advances are made or disputes in science emerge. However, stories on risk rarely become major public issues, dominating headlines for days or weeks unless they involve 'matters of state'—that is major political involvement. This can be seen by comparing the profile of coronary heart disease (CHD) with food safety, remembering that CHD kills many more people each year than food poisoning. Between January 1988 and the end of 1992 BBC television network news broadcast 128 items on food safety and between 1973 and 1991 food safety stories made the front page of the *Times* and *Sunday Times* 90 times. By contrast, CHD appeared only 25 times on BBC TV news and on the front page of the *Times* and *Sunday Times* on only ten occasions (Macintyre *et al.* 1999).

It is now commonplace for sections of the news media to report on the real and perceived motives of government communication, as in the fixation on 'spin doctors'. Here *perceived* divisions or excessive secrecy within government departments are very important. In the case of Patulin in apple juice, secrecy was a key element in the 'news value' of the story. There were a total of 41 items in the British national press on Patulin. Thirty of these were chiefly about government secrecy. In relation to *Salmonella* infection in 1988–1989 the key issue was the perceived division between MAFF and the Department of Health.

News values across the media tend to attach a high importance to controversy, division within government or between the experts, and secrecy. Plainly this is all rather galling to the prospective risk communicator, who may have little control over the wider environment within which s/he is situated. It can also be argued that the importance attached to such news values inhibits rational discussion of the communication of risk. However, there are two points that can be made here in relation to the public interest. First the self-interested pursuit of such news values as a means to maximize audiences may sometimes coincide with the public interest in making government more transparent, even if in an unintentional, distorted, or sensationalist way. Secondly, notwithstanding the pressures of the market and the tendency towards commercialism, some sections of the media retain something of a public service ethos, which may at times be helpful to government as well as on occasion obstructing its risk communication activities. However, it is clearly possible for there to be conflicting assessments of the role of the media. From the point of view of some risk communicators much media treatment of BSE in 1996 was irresponsible. However, it could equally be argued that pointing up the apparent contradiction between previous and present ministerial statements on the risks of BSE represented not so much media misbehaviour, as previous risk communication mistakes coming back to haunt the present.

We can conclude this section by noting the close interaction of the media with their sources in the production of news.

# The public

## Sources of belief

In risk analysis 'scientific' knowledge or belief is often counterposed with public or 'lay' knowledge or belief. More often the terminology used is 'scientific fact' versus public 'perception'. The problem is then located as a lack of public knowledge or understanding. This is due in some versions to 'human intellectual limitations' (Covello 1983). Curiously though, scientists, social scientists, and risk analysts (or sometimes just 'experts') are not thought to be subject to such limitations. As is clear from the rest of this volume, this type of public deficit approach has been increasingly discredited in recent years and it is certainly not supported by our own research work (Kitzinger 1990, 1993; Miller *et al.* 1998; Macintyre *et al.* 1998).

Public views are not formed from thin air. Equally they are not simply dictated by the media or ministerial pronouncements or by lay 'perspectives' or 'cultures'. Judgements are made according to the information available from the media, education, friends and family, and other sources and evaluated against previous experience and information. Experience is patterned by class, ethnicity, gender, nationality, region, and age, as well as by personal experience, and evaluated by means of logical processes. It is misleading to try to redeem public perceptions as rational without an analysis of how and why people make judgements. Trust in government is not a stable or uniform filter through which new information is strained, but varies. Although polls show trust in government as low, in fact there are times when people (even those who say they distrust the government or the media) do believe what the government tells them. It seems likely that trust is related to the specifics of the information content and the other sources that make it credible. The extent to which political disputes about risk are at the centre of public debate is important here. We can compare the public response to AIDS and BSE in this context. The significant loss of public trust over BSE was not paralleled in the case of AIDS, where a significant consensus developed that HIV was a serious threat to heterosexuals and where discrimination against so called 'high-risk groups' was discouraged. Both of these messages were widely accepted by the public. Stated trust in government may, therefore, not be a reliable indicator of public belief and response. An example from our research on food scares might illustrate the point. The respondent started by saying she didn't know much about *Salmonella* but then proceeded to rattle off the official advice about cooking eggs. When asked how she knew, she responded:

> 'I don't know really, I suppose it just seems like common sense. But ... I must have got it from somewhere ... I suppose I picked up a lot of things from the magazines that I read and there were a lot of people saying things on TV about how to cook eggs ... Isn't that funny, I just thought I'd always done that naturally' (Macintyre *et al.*, in press).

Public views are formed from a melange of influences. The media are certainly important here, but other factors also intervene in the process of opinion formation. Media information is evaluated against personal experience, according to processes of logic and against alternative infor-mation. This means that those approaches that attempt to analyse risk perception in terms of psychological tendencies such as 'optimistic bias' tend to overestimate the significance of 'public factors' in risk communication.

There is a need to examine where information and ideas come from and how these are processed, rather than assuming that events in the world are transparently available to human perception. Equally, some approaches that focus on 'lay perspectives' tend not to examine them in the context of the circulation of information and values in society. Approaches of this kind can tend towards the pessimistic in concluding that risk communication could not be much improved.

## Listening to the public

One consequence of our argument for practical improvements to risk communication is the increasing involvement of the public in setting priorities for risk management and communication. This type of procedure has already been codified in government policy in relation to the NHS aim of listening to 'local voices' (NHS Management Executive 1992) and is being tried in other areas of policy. Citizens' juries, consumer panels, consensus conferences, and their ilk are all ways of trying to incorporate public views and concerns into policy-making (and have recently been tried out in the field of 'the new genetics' and human health). Such approaches could also usefully be taken in relation to risk communication. However, there is a need to be clear about the reasons and rationale for such approaches. There is a danger that they can be used as a means of reaching and justifying a preconceived end, as has been alleged in relation to health care decisions, rather than as an open ended means of incorporating public views into decision-making (for a discussion, see Miller and Philo 1995).

# Decision-makers

The media have a clear, indirect influence on policy-making in that they can influence public beliefs and behaviour to which decision-makers then have to respond. The clearest examples are the changes in purchasing behaviour following media coverage. We are thinking here of the effect of the *Salmonella* and BSE crises in prompting a sharp drop in egg and beef sales. But we can also think of changes in behaviour over the longer term which have been intentionally prompted by government risk communication, such as the increase in sales of semi-skimmed milk and the decrease in consumption of sugar from the bowl, that were prompted by health education advice on the risks of dietary fats and sugars. Public opinion (or crucially *perceptions* of public opinion) can drive policy and decision-making and nudge decision-makers or ministers into decisions they would not otherwise have made, e.g. in the response to media coverage of shoddy slaughterhouse practice that had been ignored when raised privately by environmental health officers (Miller 1999). But policy-makers do ignore public concern on some issues, particularly if opposition is not mobilized.

Risk communicators, scientists, decision-makers, and other policy actors are members of the general public and themselves routinely consume media representations. However, the media do not just communicate with the public en masse; information is targeted by both risk communicators and journalists. There is a sense in which much political debate in the media is debate between elites, to which the rest of the public can listen in if it wishes. But there are stories in the media that are intended by those who disclose them to reach very small numbers of people, such as senior members of a particular government committee or a particular permanent secretary. Thinking about the media in this way should make it apparent that the media can play an intimate and direct role in policy-making. Moreover, policy-makers and experts have differing interests in media coverage that can have different influences on different areas. There are a number of occasions in recent history where proposed cut-backs and redundancies in scientific funding or in the staffing of government bodies have been put on hold or reversed following news coverage of particular risks (e.g. issues such as AIDS and the 'flesh-eating bug', both of which had consequences for risk assessment and surveillance personnel at, for example, the Public Health Laboratory Service). Holding onto staff who would otherwise have been made redundant can even occur when the organization has done its best to play down the significance of a particular scare, such as in the case of the flesh-eating bug.


# The resolution of public issues

Public issues decline when there is some sort of resolution of the perceived problem in the public arena. This does not mean that the problem itself is necessarily addressed, simply that the contradictions which made the story news are resolved. Thus, in relation to *Salmonella*, the departure of Edwina Currie and the compensation granted to producers, together with a reorientation in the media which blamed consumers rather than producers, killed the story. *Salmonella* Enteritidis PT4 poisoning, however, has continued to rise. By contrast, the first emergence of BSE as a public issue in 1990 was only partially resolved with the result that it returned to the public agenda periodically between 1990 and 1995, and then spectacularly in March 1996.

# Concluding remarks

At the methodological level, risk communication research needs to do more than simply examine the media or the public. It needs to examine the activities of all the actors engaged in the circuit of risk communication and crucially the relations between them. At present there is a rather heavy concentration on investigating public 'perceptions', 'attitudes', or 'perspectives'. This needs to be complemented by a much greater investment in the other parts of the circuit and in examining the relations between public beliefs and the rest of the circuit of communication. One of the most neglected areas of research in our view is the process by which risk communication campaigns are planned and executed. It seems to us that this would repay serious investigation by social scientists.

How risks are communicated depends on the relationships between the four sets of actors outlined in this paper, and not on the objective severity of any given risk. The relationship is unstable and in flux, so it is not possible to predict exactly which risks will be taken up on the public agenda and given extensive exposure. Nor are public reactions straightforwardly predictable. However, it is possible to understand the factors that lead to the emergence and decline of particular types of issue. This means that some measure of 'foresight' may be attainable. Furthermore, given that there are identifiable factors that influence the emergence of public issues, it is possible, though likely to be very difficult, to change the ways in which science, policy, the media, and the public interact.

## REFERENCES

Acheson, D. (1992). Behold a pale horse: a view from Whitehall. *PHLS Microbiology Digest*, **10**, 133–40.

Covello, V. (1983).The perception of technological risks: a literature review. *Technological Forecasting and Social Change*, **23**, 285–97.

Farrant, W. and Russell, J. (1986). *The Politics of health information: beating heart disease as a case study in the production of Health Education Council publications*. Bedford Way Papers No. 28, Institute of Education, London.

Kitzinger, J. (1990). Audience understandings of AIDS media messages: a discussion of methods. *Sociology of Health and Illness*, **12**, 319–35.

Kitzinger, J. (1993). Understanding AIDS—media messages and what people know about Acquired Immune Deficiency Syndrome. In *Getting the message,* (ed. J. Eldridge), pp. 271–304. Routledge, London.

Macintyre, S., Reilly, J., Miller, D., and Eldridge, J. (1998). Food, choice, food scares and health: the role of the media. In *The Nation's diet*, (ed. A. Murcott). Addison, Wesley, Longman, Harlow.

Miller, D. (1995). Introducing the 'gay gene': media and scientific representations. *Public Understanding of Science*, **4**, 264–84.

Miller, D. (1999). Risk, science and policy: definitional struggles, information management and the media. *Social Science and Medicine* special edition 'Science speaks to policy'. In press.

Miller, D. and Philo, G. (1995). *Communicating change in the NHS: A review of health communication campaigns, media coverage of health care issues and the process of public opinion and belief formation.* Report for the Communication Directorate of the NHS Executive, Leeds.

Miller, D. and Reilly, J. (1995). Making an issue of food safety: the media, pressure groups and the public sphere. In *Eating agendas: food, eating and nutrition as social problems*, (ed. D. Maurer and J. Sobal), pp. 305–36. Aldine De Gruyter, New York.

Miller, D., Kitzinger, J., Williams, K., and Beharrell, P. (1998). *The circuit of mass communication: media strategies, representation and audience reception in the AIDS crisis.* Sage, London.

NHS Management Executive (1992). *Local voices: the views of local people in purchasing for health*. Department of Health, London.

# 19 Improving risk communication: scenario-based workshops

Simon French and John Maule

*School of Informatics, University of Manchester* and
*Leeds University Business School, University of Leeds*

## Summary

This chapter describes the design and delivery of a series of training workshops for the Department of Health. As set out in Chapter 16, these formed part of a wider programme to develop the Department's communication strategies on public risk in relation to health issues. Each workshop was based around a hypothetical scenario which was developed further during the day. Activities alternated between exploring responses to issues within the scenario and presentations on research findings from behavioural, sociological, and psychological studies on risk communication and perception. The workshops were well received and have played a role in developing the Department's communication of health risks.

## Introduction

The philosophy of (public) language stemming from Wittgenstein's 'language games' and Searle's speech acts emphasizes that an utterance or piece of writing is an act in a 'game of interactions' (Wittgenstein 1953; Searle 1969). From this standpoint the primary purpose of the spoken or written word is to engender a change in the behaviour of the recipient, rather than the transfer of information. While we do not wish to become involved in philosophical debates about the foundations of language, we do commend this perspective as a very useful one in thinking about risk communication and the development of strategies for informing the public about health risks.

We recognize that any communication of a health risk should be ethical, providing the public with an honest and an unbiased assessment of the risk and any preventative or precautionary measure that might be necessary. However, we find it helpful to remember that any communication is an act in a 'language game' with the public. In order to take the decision to commit to that act, the public body concerned should recognize that the act will have a variety of consequences for different stakeholder groups. There is some advantage, therefore, in structuring the development of public statements, their timing, and content as a decision process that can benefit from the application of many management techniques used to support other kinds of decisions.

In the following we describe some developmental workshops which were run within the Department of Health. The primary purpose of these workshops was to sensitize those charged with public risk communication to the issues involved and to provide them with some simple tools to help in structuring the decision process. Early on, we realized that any didactic instruction based upon a 'chalk-and-talk' approach would be ineffective. First, to learn to use tools one needs to use them. Secondly, we were not confident in our own knowledge of all the issues that we should introduce for discussion. The participants in the workshops had a wide range of backgrounds and professional responsibilities, were from central and regional offices, and included staff from the Press Office and those responsible for formulating and communicating policy. They already had a wealth of practical experience of risk communication from their day-to-day work activities. We needed a mechanism to capitalize upon this experience and to enable them to share their own knowledge and experience, as well as inject advice from our own perspectives and expertise. Accordingly, we focused each workshop on a hypothetical scenario involving many aspects of risk communication, alternating between activities directed at developing a communication strategy for the scenario and presentations on background material from the workshop leaders.

The organization of this paper may suggest rather more foresight and rationality in the design of the workshops than was, in fact, present. We developed them through prototyping, beginning with an afternoon session before progressing to five full-day workshops. The material and the emphases we placed upon different aspects evolved as we discovered strengths and weaknesses in the background and working behaviour of the participants. None the less, we believe it more useful to those who will develop future workshops to explain their organization in a more structured form.

The workshops were designed and presented by a team consisting of the authors, Peter Bennett and David Coles, from the Department of Health and Lisa Simpson from the University of Leeds. We fully acknowledge their contribution and see our role in this paper as reporting the work of this larger team rather than claiming any originality ourselves.

In the next section we describe the material that we sought to convey and the management science tools that we recommended for structuring the decision process. In later sections we describe the organization of the workshops and give examples of the scenarios that we used.

# Material covered in the workshops

It is useful to categorize the material we sought to convey into two general headings similar to those set out in Chapter 16:

> *context knowledge*: *viz.* public perception and assessment of risk, based on findings from behavioural, psychological, and sociological studies which suggest how the public may react to risk communication strategies.

> *process skills*: *viz.* management science techniques that may be used to structure decision processes and catalyse creative thought.

## Public perception and assessment of risk

The primary aims here were (i) to introduce participants to contemporary theory and research on risk perception and communication, and (ii) in the context of the hypothetical risk scenario, to show how this body of knowledge can increase their understanding of how the public is likely to react to risks, and how this should inform communication strategies.

The formal input was delivered in two separate sections. The first section, the *individual context*, focused on the thinking processes that can lead to error and bias on the part of individual 'experts' and members of the public alike (see Chapter 1 and, in more depth, Kahneman *et al.* 1982, Baron 1994, Bazerman 1998; Dawes 1988). Effects such as anchoring, availability, poor and illusory framing, ignoring base rates, misconceptions of randomness, poor calibration, and over-confidence were all covered. The need to seek feedback to calibrate judgement and contrary evidence to avoid the danger of 'confirmation bias' were highlighted as simple but valuable ways of improving individual judgement and, when adopted across groups, of improving organizational effectiveness.

Non-probabilistic influences on risk judgements were reviewed, based on the research developed from within the psychometric paradigm (Slovic 1987). These were summarized in the series of fright factors set out in Chapter 1, whose presence or absence could critically determine the strength and direction of public responses to risks. These were used to predict likely responses to the hypothetical scenario, and the implications of this for management and communication strategies. Consistent with our views described above, the existence of fright factors emphasizes that acts of communication engender changes in behaviour of the recipient in addition to any transfer of information. One of the reasons that man learnt to communicate was to convey warnings. 'Ugh! Ugh! Aargh!', although graphic, was not a particularly precise way of warning others that a sabre-toothed tiger had wandered into the far end of the cave. One of the purposes served by an evolving language was to locate and identify threats, and prepare others to face them. For the threats faced as language evolved, being frightened was a very effective response. Fright is a biological state in which the body's systems are configured specifically for the purposes of flight, and flight was usually the most effective strategy. Our language still has words that engender fright, even if for today's threats flight may be neither a sensible nor a feasible course of action. For instance, in a number of contraceptive pill scares, the 'flight' response for the women concerned has been to stop taking the pill, which exposed them to higher health risks from pregnancy or terminations. Also, there is much evidence that in the region around Chernobyl many of the health problems experienced by the local population are related to stress rather than directly to the increased environmental radiation arising from the nuclear accident in 1986 (Karao-glou *et al.* 1995). It is important, therefore, to appreciate which words are likely to carry a vestigial fright and flight response (Covello 1991).

The second section of the course focused on the *social context* (Kasperson and Stallen 1991), briefly reviewing two contemporary theories, *Cultural Theory* and *Social Amplification Theory*, each discussed in Part I of this volume (especially Chapters 3 and 5, respectively). Cultural theory was used to highlight the importance of recognizing that society is composed of different groups, each with distinctive world-views, and each likely to perceive and act differently in the face of risk. Social amplification theory provided the context for discussing factors likely to intensify public reactions to risks. Special emphasis was placed on the amplifying role of the media, and a list of *media triggers* was presented, highlighting the features likely to stimulate media interest. These factors were used to discuss the likely media response to the hypothetical risk scenario. Finally, the importance of trust was discussed and factors enhancing trust identified (Renn and Levine 1991). These were briefly reviewed in the context of the Department's current practices.

Both sections of the course grounded material in the context of the hypothetical risk scenario, and concluded with a summary identifying the implications of the material presented for improving risk communication.

## Decision process skills

We were aware from discussions with members of the Department that there was little, if any, formal structuring of processes involved in designing a risk communication strategy for a health issue. In many cases, the Department acted in a reactive mode to media stories or press releases of other organizations. Even when it had control of the agenda, there was little recognition that strategic development requires both process and context expertise. While it attempted to deploy much of the latter, there was little attempt to focus on the generic processes. We therefore sought to:

(1) sensitize the participants to the value of thinking strategically and attending to the *process* of developing a risk communication strategy in addition to addressing the specific health issues in a particular case;

(2) provide the participants with simple 'pencil and paper' tools which they might use quickly to help them think about the issues involved in a particular case.

One fact that we were slow to appreciate, but were addressing with almost every second breath by the end of the series of workshops, was that the Department lacked a culture of thinking about *objectives* in dealing with communication. We believe that *value-focused thinking* (Keeney 1992) is a key attitude of mind for dealing with any strategic matter. To quote Keeney (1992, p. 3)

'Values are what we care about. As such, values should be the driving force for our decision making. They should be the basis for the time and effort we spend thinking about decisions. But this is not the way it is. It is not even close to the way it is.'

'Instead, decision making usually focuses on the choice among alternatives. Indeed, it is common to characterise a decision problem by the alternatives available. It seems as if the alternatives present themselves and the decision problem begins when at least two alternatives have appeared. Descriptively, I think this represents almost all decision situations. Prescriptively, it should be possible to do much better'.

There are clear advantages in value-focused thinking. First, it is a more creative way of working. Thinking too much about alternatives seems to constrain the mind, holding its attention on what initially seems possible and what seems to bound the possible. Thinking first about the ultimate objectives opens up the mind and allows it to think along lines such as 'I wish ...' or 'why can't we ...', leading to a more imaginative range of actions from which to choose. Secondly, it directs attention to what matters and makes it easier to avoid wasting time on superfluous or irrelevant detail. Thirdly, there are also advantages in relation to team building, implementation, and communication because one is clear about what one is trying to achieve.

Thus, one of the key messages we sought to convey was the need to be clear about objectives and continually check that the developing (risk communication) strategy addresses them. We also provided training in more specific strategic management tools and concepts such as:

- simple methods for *identifying stakeholders* and their degree of influence, for *identifying uncertainties* and their importance, and for monitoring how these may change over time
- the idea of *robustness* (Rosenhead 1978), i.e. the need to be 'roughly right' rather than 'precisely wrong' and hence to design strategies leaving later options open
- the qualitative use of *decision trees* (Wells 1982) to develop a richer and more contingent understanding of problems.

Decision trees and robustness were introduced partly to open up discussion of the value of thinking contingently. In addition, the importance of anticipating the responses of other stakeholders and generally 'thinking ahead' were discussed as a means of helping the Department develop strategies for keeping control of the agenda. In this respect we also very briefly introduced some of the ideas coming to the fore in the current scenario planning literature (van der Heijden 1996).

## The workshops

The programme for a typical workshop is given in Table 19.1. Note that the precision of the timings is entirely illusory. We felt that a timetable provided the participants and presenters with some comfort of control and organization. In practice, each day evolved according to the interests and experiences of the participants, with continual rescheduling of sessions.

## Scenarios and their development

In running this programme of workshops, seven scenarios were developed. Six were used and one actually happened before we could use it! A summary of one scenario used is given in Box 19.1 below.

---

**Box 19.1    Hypothetical scenario: Condoms and cancer**

---

(Phase 1) The Department of Health is contacted by the Department of Medical Statistics at a London University college about a longitudinal study into men's health, focusing on their contraceptive practices and financed by an AIDS charity, a condom manufacturer, and a research council. Analysis of the first five years' data has thrown up significant evidence of a link between prostate cancer and the use of condoms, apparently related to the commonly used spermicide Nonoxynol-9.

Realizing the potential significance of this result, the principal investigator leading the study has arranged for a colleague in Scotland to review the methodology informally. She has found no flaws in it. The next normal step would be to submit the report for peer review and publication. However, the researchers are forewarning the Department and are willing to take any reasonable and responsible cause of action.

*What should be done? What advice should be sought? Who should be briefed?*

(Phase 2) A research student involved in the investigation refuses to honour the confidentiality agreement he has signed. He feels very strongly that the risk of prostate cancer should be in the public domain. His view relates to a strong religious belief and an abhorrence of promiscuity. Meanwhile, both the charity and the manufacturer concerned have argued against going public on the finding until alternative supplies of condoms are available. This will take weeks to arrange, and other spermicides are also less effective.

(Phase 3) The *Sunday Telegraph* prints a story on the study. It is responsible and does suggest that use of a condom is preferable to unprotected sex. However, it also carries an article by the student's church group leader, taking a fundamentalist Christian stance. The TV and radio morning programmes have all carried the story and it was heavily discussed between religious leaders on *Frost at Breakfast*.

The Department of Health is being approached by all media for a statement. What line should be taken?

---

**Table 19.1**  Programme of a typical workshop

| Programme | | Objectives and content of session |
|---|---|---|
| 9.00–9.15: | Coffee | |
| 9.15–9.30: | Introduction | Aims of the day, structure, and ground rules |
| *Scenario Phase 1 introduced* | | |
| 9.30–9.50: | Participants split into groups to prepare immediate response (identify three questions they would ask and what their next actions would be) | |
| 9.50–10.15: | Plenary to compare and contrast immediate responses | Response to Phase 1 of scenario |
| 10.15–10.40: | Presentation: *Structuring methods I* | Different stakeholders, problem representations, uncertainties and threats<br>Strategy and tactics, uncertainties caused by 'states of the world' and actions of specific stakeholders. |
| *Scenario Phase 2 introduced* | | |
| 10.45–11.00: | *Coffee* | |
| 11.00–11.30: | Work in groups on<br>• classifying uncertainties<br>• identifying stakeholders | (Facilitators join groups to guide activities) |
| 11.30–12.00: | Plenary session. | Note unknowns and stakeholders: similarities and differences between groups |
| 12.00–12.30: | Presentation: *Public perception and assessment of risk: The individual perspective* | A review of research on how individuals perceive and act in the face of risk |
| 12.30–12.45: | Groups list key elements of their risk communication strategy | What do they see as their objectives? Who are they planning to communicate with? How to engage with key stakeholders? |
| 12.45–1.15: | Lunch | |
| 1.15–1.35: | Plenary: groups present 'strategic issues' and compare | |
| 1.35–1.55: | Presentation: *Structuring methods II* | More on the need to be clear on objectives. Scenarios as pictures of 'possible futures' driven by actions and uncertainties. Structuring decisions and events, e.g. using decision trees. |
| *Scenario Phase 3 introduced* | | |
| 2.00–2.30: | Generating contrasting scenarios. | Work in original groups, with facilitators. Produce *one good and two contrasting bad* scenarios. |
| 2.30–3.00: | Groups report back to plenary | Note differences between groups' representations and implications of these: insights provided by structuring approach. |

| | | |
|---|---|---|
| 3.00–3.30: | Presentation and discussion: *Public perception and assessment of risk: The social perspective 1* | A review of social theories, identification of media triggers and a discussion of the importance of trust. During this presentation one facilitator takes some of the developing scenario material and produces some draft decision trees |
| 3.00–3.45: | Tea | |
| 3.45–4.00: | *Presentation of outline decision tree structures* | Rough decision tree structure, note some pros and cons of different outcomes.<br>Idea of multiple criteria and how analysis can be taken further. |
| 4.00–4.30: | Consider and discuss a draft press release and work in groups to draft messages: Groups produce notes summarizing intended communications. Reconsider communication strategy and tactics in light of all material introduced so far. | |
| 4.30–5.00: | Presentation of draft messages and discussion | Report back on group activity: compare and contrast responses. Reprise:<br>• guidelines on risk communication<br>• risk communication within the policy process uses and sources of further analysis<br>• comments on the workshop |

There are some points to note. First, the scenario is entirely hypothetical. In particular, we know of no reason to suspect/implicate Nonoxynol-9 in any health risk relating to prostrate cancer. Secondly, the description here differs from the one used in the workshop in one respect only. In the workshop we named a specific statistics group at a London college, a condom manufacturer, and a charity group to help the participants role play. For similar reasons, in the discussion within the workshop we also related the story line to other current happenings in the media and changes happening as the new Labour government took control.

During the workshops we learnt much about developing interesting scenarios. We found that it stimulated discussion greatly if we confounded the health risk issues with other factors that necessitated interaction with other government departments or which would capture disproportionate media interest. The scenario described above involves important religious and moral issues that are likely to become part of the public and media debate. In another, there were international aspects which involved a need to work with the Foreign Office. In others we introduced other fright factors, e.g. by directing the risk at children. Simpson (1998) discusses scenario generation further.

In the afternoons of the early workshops we asked the participants to draft a press release. However, we found that in doing so they quickly fell back into old ways and old forms of words which did not reflect the ideas that we had been seeking to convey. In the later workshops we prompted this drafting phase by first presenting a press release for criticism and asking them to improve it. In Box 19.2 below we give the draft used to prompt discussion for the scenario described above. It should be emphasized that these draft releases were intended to stimulate discussion and were not offered as examples of good practice. We were aware of many flaws and hostages to fortune in the manner in which they were worded. It is perhaps a comment on the complexity of the issue that we failed to identify ourselves all the criticisms that were levelled within the workshop!

---

**Box 19.2    Condoms and cancer: draft press release**

---

The Department has been aware of the results of the study since last Thursday, 29 May. It has been examining their implications and taking expert advice on how to proceed upon what are, after all, preliminary results. None the less, the Department would emphasize that it is taking this issue very seriously and does not expect the results of the study to be refuted by further analysis.

Prostate cancer is very common. Estimates suggest that one-third of older men have signs of the cancer, but that it is seldom the cause of their ultimate death. The link with the spermicide in question would, it is estimated, account for about 80–100 deaths per annum from this cause—a very small risk for the British population given the risk of HIV infection through the practice of less-safe sex or the risk to female partners of some of the alternative forms of contraception. There is no empirical evidence of a risk from Nonoxynol-9 when it is used in pessaries.

The Department does not wish to enter into a debate upon morality, which is in any case outside its remit. It does, however, confirm that complete abstinence from promiscuous relationships will remove all risks associated with HIV and the spermicide concerned.

---

# Conclusions and future prospects

The programme of workshops was intended to raise awareness of relevant research, to promote earlier and more systematic attention to these issues, but to avoid any impression of peddling easy answers. In developing and presenting them, we ourselves have also been engaged in a learning process. For example, we have been led to increase the emphasis on certain process issues—notably the need for clear objectives and the importance of review.

All events were well received, with positive feedback from questionnaire evaluation. All participants enjoyed the events, learned from them, and thought them valuable. It is interesting to note what they thought were the most important issues that they would take away from the workshops. The following list summarizes their responses in answer to this question.

Setting clear communication objectives.

Understanding how the public perceives risks.

There is a gap between quantitative statements (professions) and qualitative statements (public), and a need for appropriate terminology.

Use public to educate profession.

Use of decision trees to think ahead. Analyse potential consequences of taking different lines rather than only considering how likely your information is to be correct.

Keeping control of the communication agenda.

Reactive versus proactive responses.

Robustness—don't get painted into a corner.

Use of thinking tools and checklists, and remembering to use them.

Identifying stakeholders.

Audit and review performance.

Need for strong internal communications.

Keeping track of the wider picture.

Whose risk? What risk? Keeping track of this and how it is perceived.

Within the wider programme outlined in Chapter 16, it is intended to continue with developmental workshops as an established part of staff training. Further events are planned, one proposal being to allow both Departmental staff and representatives of other stakeholders to react to risk scenarios. Another aim is to develop further generic guidance: one perceived need is for a set of 'templates' characterizing risk communication issues and offering material relevant to each. Designing such material in a way that can be supported by credible research is a major undertaking.

To summarize, we have developed a style of workshop that seeks to help health officials address issues of risk communication. While we do not believe we can provide a single 'correct' set of guidelines, some key principles seem to be gaining wide acceptance. We agree that three of the most important are those set out in the Preface to Part 4 above and in the Chief Medical Officer's Annual Report (Department of Health 1997):

1.  While public reactions to statements about risk can seem surprising, they are not totally unpredictable.

2.  Effective communication is necessarily a two-way process.

3.  Good risk communication requires a coherent strategy, rather than ad hoc reaction to events.

If the workshops convey no more than this, we could do worse.

## REFERENCES

Baron, J. (1994). *Thinking and deciding* (2nd edn). Cambridge University Press, Cambridge.

Bazerman, M. (1998). *Managerial decision-making* (4th edn). John Wiley and Sons, Chichester.

Covello, V. T. (1991). Risk comparisons and risk communication: issues and problems in comparing health and environmental risks. In *Communicating risks to the public: international perspectives*. (ed. R. E. Kasperson and P. M. J. Stallen), pp. 79–124. Kluwer, Dordrecht.

Dawes, R. (1988). *Rational choice in an uncertain world.* Harcourt Brace Jovanovich, San Diego.

Department of Health (1997). *Chief Medical Officer's Annual Report (1996).* Department of Health, London.

Kahneman, D., Slovic, P., and Tversky, A. (ed.) (1982). *Judgement under uncertainty.* Cambridge University Press, Cambridge.

Karaoglou, A., Desmet, G., Kelly, G. N., and Menzel, H. G. (ed.) (1995). *The radiological consequences of the Chernobyl accident.* EUR 16544 EN. CEC, Luxembourg.

Kasperson, R. E. and Stallen, P. M. J. (ed.) (1991). *Communicating risks to the public: international perspectives.* Kluwer, Dordrecht.

Keeney, R. L. (1992). *Value-focused thinking.* Harvard University Press, Boston, Mass.

Rosenhead, J. (1978). An education in robustness. *Journal of Operational Research Society,* **29**, 105–11.

Scarle, J. R. (1969). *Speech acts: an essay in the philosophy of language.* Cambridge University Press, Cambridge.

Slovic, P. (1987). Perception of risk. *Science,* **236**, 280–5.

Simpson, L. (1998). PhD Thesis, School of Computer Studies, University of Leeds, Leeds.

van der Heijden, K. (1996). *Scenarios, the art of strategic conversation.* John Wiley and Sons, Chichester.

Wells, G. E. (1982). The use of decision analysis in the imperial group. *Journal of Operational Research Society,* **33**, 313–18.

Wittgenstein, L. (1953). *Philosophical investigations.* Basil Blackwell, Oxford.

# 20 Learning from experience: the need for systematic evaluation methods

Simon Gerrard

*Deputy Director, Centre of Environmental Risk, School of Environmental Sciences, University of East Anglia*

## Introduction

Managing risks involves the combination of several diverse components ranging from technical assessments to public perception studies and risk communication strategies. However, one of the weakest links in this chain of components is evaluation. For a variety of reasons, comprehensive evaluations are rarely conducted in the context of risk management. Often those in charge have neither the time nor the necessary resources to do more than quickly review 'progress'. Sometimes, for political reasons, those responsible may prefer not to know the detailed results of their efforts. However, with pressures on risk managers increasing, so is the premium on fully understanding why risk management interventions do and do not work.

This paper examines the role of systematic evaluation for risk communication as a means of developing better a understanding of the effectiveness of our efforts. Before considering a benchmark case study conducted by the UK Health and Safety Executive (HSE), some of the principles of systematic evaluation are discussed.

## The European risk communication network

In an attempt to address the twin problems of developing our understanding of risk communication and meeting the rising number of increasingly intensive risk management challenges, the World Health Organisation

(WHO) inspired the creation of the European Risk Communication Network (ERCN). The ERCN was asked to provide a link between academia, government, industry, and other groups involved in risk management with the broad aim of increasing the collective knowledge on risk communication issues. Since 1990 it has been working to do just that. Initially, much of the ERCN's activity has rested on the need to establish a European perspective on risk perception and communication to account more realistically for the significant differences between peoples and cultures in Europe. Lessons learned from experiences in North America have informed the development of risk communication, but their applicability in a European context is not guaranteed.

To develop a European perspective requires, in part, learning from our own experiences. The task of collecting, collating, and analysing these is one of the challenges the ERCN is currently undertaking. However, if the early days of this task have established the paucity of documentation regarding European experiences with risk communication, then they have also shed a powerful light on the considerable potential for learning—usually not realized—provided by the systematic evaluation of risk communication interventions. Ultimately, developing systematic methods of evaluation will foster the development of self-learning organizations.

# Introduction to evaluation

Evaluating the performance of a particular policy or intervention is widely recognized as a crucial aspect of effective management, yet it is an aspect often overlooked. Far too often risk management policies are developed in an uninformed manner that stems from a lack of comprehensive evaluation. Such policies are the ones that are most likely to be ineffectual. Recognizing the weaknesses as well as the strengths of policy decisions is an important step towards increasing overall effectiveness.

Evaluation is the systematic application of research procedures for assessing the conceptualization, design, implementation, and utility of interventions (Rossi and Freeman 1993). The term *intervention* is used to refer to a broad range of activities, from large-scale national and international policy initiatives to medium- and small-scale activities such as seminars and mailshots in educational campaigns. Evaluation may have several objectives, but perhaps the most common overall aim is to assess the worth of a particular action. However, evaluation theory is often applied at a macro level. Its transferability to micro levels is less well researched, yet this is the level at which the majority of risk perception and communication interventions are implemented.

## Evaluation as part of a risk management strategy

Risk management is often depicted as a linear process with a beginning—
usually hazard identification—and a end—often policy development.
Crucially, what is often underplayed by a linear approach is the role of
feedback. This is particularly relevant here as the main source of feedback comes from evaluation. Figure 20.1 adopts a cyclical view of risk
management which is less inclined to regard the process as having discrete
endpoints.

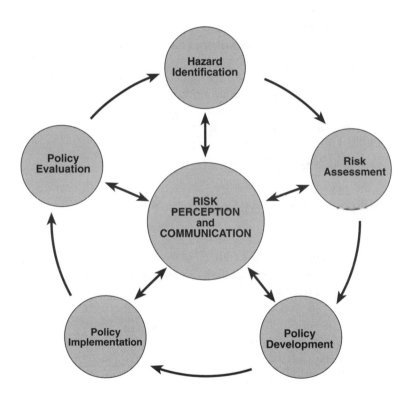

**Fig. 20.1** The risk management cycle. Risk management is often depicted as a linear
process. Ten years of research experience at the Centre of Environmental Risk
School of Environmental Sciences has shown that risk management is a cyclical
process which feeds back into itself in a series of iterative stages. This highlights the
importance of evaluation in risk management as a systematic means of learning from
previous experiences. Such evaluations are rarely conducted, yet these are the only
way in which effects can be identified and measured. Thus, effective risk management
requires that systematic evaluation is undertaken (Soby *et al.* 1993).

Though one might instinctively choose to begin at the 'top' of the cycle, there is no particular reason why this has to be the case. Indeed, the potential role of evaluation in *defining* hazards of interest is significant. Regarding risk management as a cyclical process reinforces the importance of proper evaluation as a means of providing the correct checks and balances to the ongoing development of risk management strategies. Both in the UK and the US, risk policy organizations have recently chosen to adopt a cyclical view of risk management that stresses the importance of comprehensive evaluation (Parliamentary Office of Science and Technology 1996; Presidential/Congressional Commission 1997).

## Barriers to evaluation

A number of barriers exist to frustrate comprehensive evaluation. Evaluation tends to be a very time-consuming and therefore costly part of the risk management cycle. As it tends to occur in the later stages of the cycle it is often convenient for it to be overlooked. Evaluation also has the potential to highlight poor performance. Because few risk managers really want to be shown how badly they are doing, evaluations are often more readily conducted to illustrate good performances than in situations where the results may highlight intractable problems. This is a particularly important point as it has potential impact on those undertaking evaluations. Though integral to the reliability and accuracy of the exercise, they may yet themselves be uncertain as to the motives for the evaluation or the impact of its results, and therefore conduct the evaluation in a less than adequate manner. The motives for undertaking evaluation can arouse distrust and anxiety and promote unwanted internal and external competition for an organization.

Despite these potential problems, there is no doubt that comprehensive evaluations can improve performance by informing and directing new policies and fine-tuning existing initiatives. Understanding not only whether an intervention works, but the reasons why, is important in improving efforts through time.

# Principles of systematic evaluation

Planning an evaluation should be linked closely to the design of risk communication interventions. In practice, however, many evaluations are conducted in an *ad hoc* manner with little consideration of underlying assumptions or potential variables that may influence specific changes. Such 'quick and dirty' evaluations are unlikely to help the organization improve its longer term performance and are usually associated with short-term justifications for maintaining the status quo. Within more systematic evaluations there are a number of common questions that require addressing. Table 20.1 sets out the most important. Each can be attributed to a particular stage in the evaluation and to a specific activity, though some overlap may occur between the stages depending upon the specific question posited.

## Defining objectives

Objectives can be characterized as either absolute or relative. The former require total outcomes, e.g. a mailshot to *all* residents in a specified sector or area. Conversely, relative objectives are specified in the form of standards of achievement, e.g. increasing consumer understanding of a particular health issue by 50% of the 1995 levels.

In order to evaluate an intervention it is crucial to specify clear objectives. This can be done in a number of ways, though the more specific the objective the easier it is to evaluate. First, each objective should encompass a single aim. Combining more than one aim in an objective results in problematic evaluation. If one aim is achieved but the other is not, then deciding whether the objective has been met is more difficult than it needs to be. Secondly, the use of action-oriented verbs such as 'increase' rather than less specific verbs such as 'promote' has a marked effect on the subsequent evaluation. Thirdly, attaching a quantifiable end-product or result enables the objective to be evaluated more clearly. It is also useful to specify a time-scale in which the objective will be achieved.

**Table 20.1** Typical questions within evaluation stages and their corresponding activity

| Evaluation Stage | Question | Evaluation Activity |
|---|---|---|
| **Conceptualization** | What is the nature and scope of the intervention to be evaluated? | Identification of original objectives |
| | What are the problems with the existing intervention? | Identification of existing and potential problem areas |
| | What are the possible alternative actions? | Identification of possible solutions |
| | What are the appropriate target populations? | Targeting |
| **Implementation** | Is the intervention reaching its target? | Targeting |
| **Assessment** | Is the intervention effective? | Effectiveness |
| | Is the intervention cost-effective? | Cost:benefit analysis |

Source: Rossi and Freeman 1993.

## Achieving objectives

If evaluation is an important part of intervention design, then the clear definition of objectives can assist greatly in managing an intervention (see also Chapter 19). Nay (1976, pp. 97–8) identifies three criteria that must be satisfied:

(1) specification of measurable objectives including activities, costs, and outcomes;

(2) those in charge of the intervention having the motivation, ability, and authority to manage;

(3) an internal logic through which plausible, testable assumptions link the application of resources to intervention activities, the activities to intended intervention outcomes, and the outcomes to the original objectives.

## Impact models

The requirement for internal logic has led to the development of systematic models to establish the impact of policy interventions. These attempt to translate conceptual ideas regarding the regulation, modification, and control of behaviour or conditions into hypotheses on which action can be based (Rutman 1977; Rossi and Freeman 1993). The model usually takes the form of a statement of the expected relationship(s) between an intervention and its goal. Typically, a full impact model contains three hypotheses outlined in Table 20.2.

The development of a well-defined impact model is essential for intervention design and subsequent evaluation. Figure 20.2 illustrates the structure of a potential impact model for evaluating the outcomes of risk perception and communication interventions.

**Table 20.2**  Evaluation hypotheses

| Hypothesis | Description |
| --- | --- |
| **Causal hypothesis** | What causes the problem to be treated by the intervention? The most useful causal hypotheses relate the problem to processes that interventions might affect. |
| **Intervention hypothesis** | This specifies the relationship between the intended intervention actions and the processes determined in the causal hypothesis. |
| **Action hypothesis** | This determines whether the intervention is linked to the desired outcome or whether the desired outcome has occurred by other means. |

Source: Rossi and Freeman 1993.

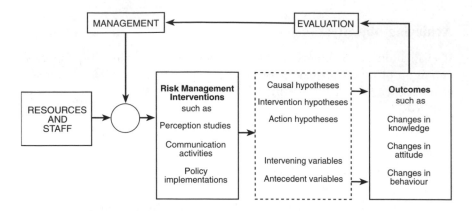

**Fig. 20.2**   Evaluation programme model (Wholey 1977, p. 45).

## Gross and net outcomes

It is important to make a distinction between gross and net outcomes, i.e. those outcomes related solely to the intervention (net) and those derived from all sources (gross). By definition, net outcomes are much more difficult to measure. One approach involves using control groups, though this is by no means straightforward. While control groups may not be affected by the risk management intervention, they may still be exposed to external factors such as news reports, court rulings, trade association initiatives, insurance interventions, and supply chain demands.

# Case study: an evaluation of risk communication techniques in UK businesses

## Background

The UK Health and Safety Executive (HSE) has responsibility for implementing, enforcing, and monitoring health and safety legislation in the UK. Traditionally, inspections at commercial and industrial premises have played a central part in discharging these responsibilities. However, as the industrial and commercial base of the UK has changed, in particular with the increase in the number of Small and Medium Enterprises (SMEs) and the changing nature and range of potential hazards, the HSE has adopted additional forms of communication including the use of mailshots and seminars. However, little is known about the effectiveness of these techniques in changing business attitudes towards health and safety matters.

In response to this lack of knowledge, the HSE has recently completed a study evaluating the effectiveness of its risk communication contact techniques. Over 6500 assessments were made in more than 1000 small firms between April 1995 and June 1997. The assessments followed a series of 43 mailshots and 22 seminar health and safety (risk) communication interventions.

## Development of aims and objectives

The stated aim of the evaluation project was:

'To find out how effective mailshots and seminars are at influencing small firms to improve their performance in important areas of health and safety in cases where they need to do so' (Health and Safely Executive 1997).

This can be regarded as the basis for the main hypothesis of the study, from which a number of sub-hypotheses were created:

Do these techniques represent value for money and a justifiable use of resources?

Are they more effective at promoting action in some sectors or on some health and safety issues than in others, and if so which?

What sort of changes are taking place: knowledge gain, improved arrangements, physical precautions?

The project attempted to identify three areas where change may occur—in **knowledge**, in **arrangements**, and in **precautions**. The choice of these variables reflected the understanding of health and safety issues in SMEs. In public-health-related risk communication interventions, changes in knowledge, arrangements, and precautions could be aligned to changes in perception and how these are linked to changes in behaviour. While we know that knowledge is not the only basis for understanding perception, evaluating changes in arrangements and precautions seems closely linked to behavioural changes that are indicative of the effectiveness of risk communication interventions.

In the terms of Table 20.2, the *causal hypothesis* links the provision of information to reasons for change, i.e. improvements in performance of the SMEs in question. Here it is important to bear in mind any antecedent variables that may have an additional influence. These include the characteristics of SMEs (such as their opportunity or ability to respond to change), the organizational cultures associated with different industrial sectors or different management styles, and the background of a particular company, e.g. its prosecution record.

The *intervention hypothesis* focused on the potential links between the specific intervention (provision of health and safety information) and changes in performance that subsequently arose. Any assumptions about the 'power' of information to stimulate change had to account for intervening variables such as the nature and range of material presented, the style of presentation, and the availability of similar information from other sources.

The *action hypothesis* related to the actual changes as measured during the evaluation. Again, attention had to be paid to antecedent and intervening variables that might influence and stimulate change other than the contact techniques themselves.

## Identifying cause and effect

HSE inspectors were asked to identify the main stimulus for any action taken or planned. This provided the basis for determining an association between any change and the agent for that change. Information regarding the prime driving forces behind change was gathered from discussion with the relevant SME manager. There were a number of difficulties associated with this approach, including the question of accurate recollection of the contact technique—particularly problematic with mailshots. This posed a significant problem for the design of the evaluation project. In order for there to have been a reasonable likelihood of change, sufficient time must have elapsed—yet as time elapsed so the accurate recollection of events diminished and data reliability decreased. It was for this reason that the HSE decided to include planned as well as existing changes.

In principle, the use of case and control groups was important if other possible causes not attributable to the contact technique were to be discounted. However, in practice a number of problems arose. Ideally case and control groups should be identical except for the one variable being tested, in this case exposure to a contact technique. In practice this was impossible, and as more and more parameters were found to differ, the significance of the control group diminished. There comes a point when the time and effort of developing a control group exceeds the value of having the group. This illustrates the general need to give the value of control groups detailed consideration during the design of evaluation programmes.

## Data consistency and reliability: using formal guidance

In principle it is possible to increase reliability by improving the coordination of evaluation. Efforts were made by HSE project staff to promote a more formal approach to the pre-evaluation period by encouraging short briefing seminars/discussions with inspectors prior to the contact technique project to clarify the purpose of the evaluation. These offered an important opportunity for questions to be raised and answered.

The result was a greater understanding of, and commitment to, the evaluation process—thereby counteracting the likelihood of inconsistencies in data collection through factors such as distrust, anxiety, and low morale.

Important guidance was prepared for the HSE inspectors as to how to conduct the evaluation. On the whole this was well received, and the majority of responses received supported the view that without the guidance the evaluation would have been impossible. Although relatively complicated, the guidance was appreciated and understood by many of the contact technique evaluation project leaders. There is obviously a fine balance between providing adequate guidance to enable inspectors to complete the evaluation correctly, and overloading already busy staff with extra paperwork. Guidance needs to be clear and flexible, and sometimes produced in different forms for different purposes.

## Action, inaction, and the relationship between standards and action

In drawing any conclusions about the effectiveness of the contact technique, it was important to focus on the proportions of assessments that were associated with subsequent change. The systematic approach to evaluation enabled some important information to be gathered about the relationship between existing standards and action taken. This was particularly important as it provided a basis for justifying performance in terms of both the *quantity* and *quality* of changes stimulated by the contact techniques.

The evaluation project was able to confirm the conventional wisdom that seminars were more effective than mailshots in triggering change. However, where change was stimulated by mailshots that change tended to be more likely to be raising standards to an appropriate level. This rather surprising result has enabled the HSE to reflect carefully on the use of seminars and mailshots which would not have necessarily been the case had the evaluation measured only the quantity of change.

# Conclusions

## Quantitative and qualitative approaches—the need for triangulation

The HSE evaluation project took over two years to complete and has expended a significant level of resources. In some respects it has created more questions than answers, though the answers it has provided are proving to be very useful. Despite this, it is unlikely that this type of project could be repeated to the same degree in the near future.

As systematic evaluation becomes a more central part of everyday organizational behaviour, so its costs will be considered less significant. However, in the short term there is a pressing need to find ways to reduce costs. Combining quantitative and qualitative information may provide a ready solution. In the vast majority of cases this will improve understanding the reality of risk communication interventions. This raises an interesting issue of whether triangulation can both improve the robustness of the evaluation results and reduce the cost of developing, implementing, and analysing systematic evaluation.

A first step towards this endpoint might be for organizations to reflect carefully on the kinds of data already collected, how those collection systems might be refined to include relevant evaluation data, and how the data collected might best be used. This could be the initial basis for developing some form of audit mechanism based around a systematic evaluation of risk communication interventions.

A second important step that systematic evaluation forces risk communicators to take is to specify the measurable goals of the intervention clearly at the outset. While this may appear to be an obvious step, it is often overlooked (see also Chapter 19). Asking about the basic purpose of risk communication, how that links to our understanding of risk perception, and how we intend to achieve the desired effect is fundamental to the design, implementation, and success of risk communication and risk management interventions.

There are some striking parallels here with the conduct of epidemiological studies, and it may be that this field could provide some useful insights into the development of the evaluation of risk communication. As with epidemiology, systematic evaluation may not always be able to deliver comprehensive answers, but without asking the key questions we will surely never move forward.

---

## REFERENCES

---

Gerrard, S. P. (1995). Environmental risk management. In *Environmental sciences for environmental management*, (ed. T. O'Riordan), pp. 296–316. Longman, London.
Health and Safety Executive (1997). *Guidance for national project to evaluate contact techniques: seminars/workshops*. Internal memorandum. Health and Safety Executive, Bootle, Merseyside.

Nay, J. I. (1976). If you don't care where you get to then it doesn't matter which way you go. In *The evaluation of social interventions*, (ed. C. C. Abt). Sage, Beverley Hills, California.

Parliamentary Office of Science and Technology (1996). *Safety in numbers? Risk assessment in environmental protection.* POST, House of Commons, Millbank, London.

Presidential/Congressional Commission on Risk Assessment and Risk Management (1997). *Framework for environmental and health risk management*, Vol. 1. National Academy of Sciences, Washington DC.

Rossi, P. H. and Freeman, H. E. (1993). *Evaluation: a systematic approach*, 5th edn. Sage, London.

Rutman, L. (ed.) (1977). *Evaluation research methods: a basic guide*. Sage, Beverley Hills, California.

Soby, B. A., Simpson, A. C. D., and Ives, D. P. (1993). *Integrating public and scientific judgements into a tool kit for managing food-related risks, Stage I: Literature review and feasibility study.* CERM Research Report No. 16, University of East Anglia, Norwich.

Wholey, J. S. (1977). Evaluability assessment. In *Evaluation research methods: a basic guide*, (ed. L. Rutman), pp. 41–56. Sage, Beverley Hills, California.

# Index

uncertainty 69, 125
and
plan
and
usable i

value-focused thinking 245–6
values 7–8, 147–9, 245–6
veterinary medicines 124–6

Veterinary Medicines Directorate 124–5
visual impact media trigger 17, 89

Combined Centres for Public
Health 108, 111
willingness to pay studies 45–7

yeast, genetically modified 141–2
'yuk' factor 143